HE 251

HE 251

Community and Public Health Issues
Portland Community College

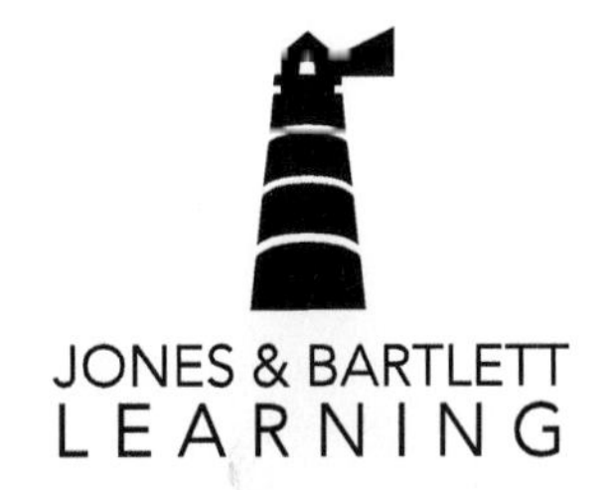

World Headquarters
Jones & Bartlett Learning
5 Wall Street
Burlington, MA 01803
978-443-5000
info@jblearning.com
www.jblearning.com

Jones & Bartlett Learning books and products are available through most bookstores and online booksellers. To contact Jones & Bartlett Learning directly, call 800-832-0034, fax 978-443-8000, or visit our website, www.jblearning.com.

This book is produced through PUBLISH – a custom publishing service offered by Jones & Bartlett Learning. For more information on PUBLISH, contact us at 800-832-0034 or visit our website at www.jblearning.com.

Disclaimer
This publication is sold with the understanding that the publisher is not engaged in rendering medical, legal, accounting, or other professional services. If medical, legal, accounting, or other professional service advice is required, the service of a competent professional should be sought. The authors, editor, and publisher have designed this publication to provide accurate information with regard to the subject matter covered. However, they are not responsible for errors, omissions, or for any outcomes related to the use of the contents of this publication and make no guarantee and assume no responsibility or liability for the use of the products and procedures described, or the correctness, sufficiency, or completeness of stated information, opinions, or recommendations. Treatments and side effects described in this publication are not applicable to all people; required dosages and experienced side effects will vary among individuals. Drugs and medical devices discussed herein are controlled by the Food and Drug Administration (FDA) and may have limited availability for use only in research studies or clinical trials. Research, clinical practice, and government regulations often change accepted standards. When consideration is being given to the use of any drug in the clinical setting, the health care provider or reader is responsible for determining FDA status of the drug, reading the package insert, and reviewing prescribing information for the most current recommendations on dose, precautions, and contraindications and for determining the appropriate usage for the product. This is especially important in the case of drugs that are new or seldom used. Any references in this publication to procedures to be employed when rendering emergency care to the sick and injured are provided solely as a general guide; other or additional safety measures might be required under particular circumstances. This publication is not intended as a statement of the standards of care required in any particular situation; circumstances and the physical conditions of patients can vary widely from one emergency to another. This publication is not intended in any way to advise emergency personnel concerning their legal authority to perform the activities or procedures discussed. Such local determination should be made only with the aid of legal counsel. Some images in this publication feature models; these models do not necessarily endorse, represent, or participate in the activities represented in the images.

Cover Image: © AbleStock

6048
Printed in the United States of America
16 15 14 13 12 10 9 8 7 6 5 4 3 2 1

PCC - Cascade Campus
Math, Science, Health & PE Division
Phone: 971-722 -5209
Fax: 971-722-5257

FAX

Pages:

To:

Fax:

Date:

Re:

From:

Fax: 971-722-5257

Phone: 971-722-5209

Cc:

Comments:

- [ ] Urgent
- [ ] For Review
- [ ] Please Comment
- [ ] Please Reply
- [ ] Please Recycle

Contents

FOUNDATIONS OF COMMUNITY HEALTH

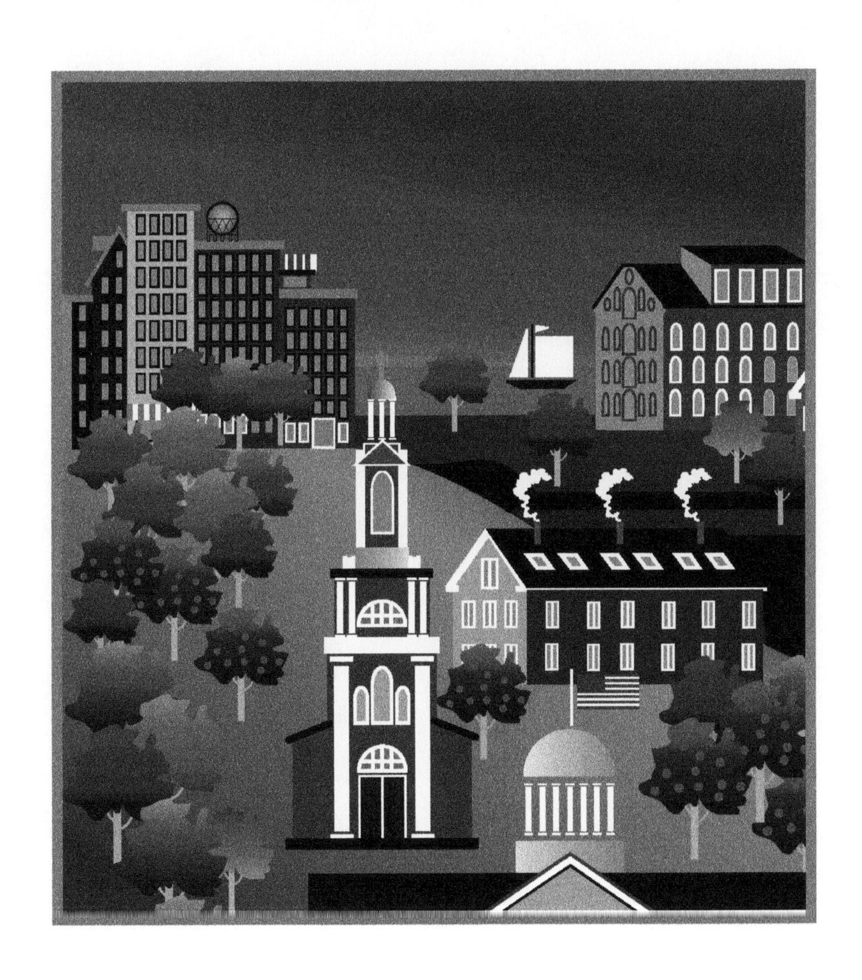

Community Health: Yesterday, Today, and Tomorrow

Chapter Outline

Scenario

Introduction
Definitions • Factors That Affect the Health of a Community

A Brief History of Community and Public Health
Earliest Civilizations • The Eighteenth Century • The Nineteenth Century • The Twentieth Century

Outlook for Community Health in the Twenty-First Century
World Planning for the Twenty-First Century • The United States' Planning for the Twenty-First Century

Chapter Summary

Scenario: Analysis and Response

Review Questions

Activities

Community Health on the Web

References

Chapter Objectives

After studying this chapter, you will be able to:

1. Accurately define the terms *health, community, community health, population health, public health, public health system,* and *global health*.
2. Briefly describe the five major determinants of health.
3. Explain the difference between personal and community health activities.
4. List and discuss the factors that influence a community's health.
5. Briefly relate the history of community/public health, including the recent U.S. history of community and public health in the twentieth and early twenty-first centuries.
6. Provide a brief overview of the current health status of Americans.
7. Describe the major community health problems facing the United States today.
8. Describe the status of efforts to improve world health and list some plans for the future.
9. Describe the purpose of the *Healthy People 2020* goals and objectives as they apply to the planning process of the health of Americans.

SCENARIO

Amy and Eric are a young working couple who are easing into a comfortable lifestyle. They have good-paying jobs, drive nice cars, are buying a home in a good neighborhood, and have two healthy preschool children. When Amy picked her children up from day care earlier in the day she learned from the head teacher that another parent had reported that his child was diagnosed with hepatitis. This news frightened Amy and made her begin to question the quality of the day care center. Amy told Eric of this situation when he got home from work. As the couple discussed whether or not they should take their children to day care as usual the following day, they discovered that they have many unanswered questions. How serious is hepatitis? What is the likelihood that their children will be at serious risk for getting the disease? What steps are being taken to control the outbreak? Is any state or local agency responsible for standardizing health practices at private day care centers in the community? Does the city, county, or state carry out any type of inspection when they license these facilities? And, if the children do not attend day care, which parent will stay home with them?

INTRODUCTION

In looking back over the last 100-plus years, it is easy to point to the tremendous progress that was made in the health and life expectancy of those in the United States (see Box 1) and of many people of the world. Infant mortality dropped, many of the infectious diseases have been brought under control, and better family planning became available. However, there is still room for improvement! Individual health behaviors, such as the use of tobacco, poor diet, and physical inactivity, have given rise to an unacceptable number of cases of illness and death from noninfectious diseases such as cancer, diabetes, and heart disease. New and emerging infectious diseases, such as the 2009 H1N1 flu and those caused by drug-resistant pathogens, are stretching resources available to control them. And events stemming from natural disasters such as floods and hurricanes, and humanmade disasters such as the Gulf oil spill and terrorism around the world have caused us to refocus our priorities. All of these events have severely disrupted Americans' sense of security[1] and sense of safety in the environment. In addition, many of these events revealed the vulnerability of the United States' ability to respond to such circumstances and highlighted the need for improvement in emergency response preparedness and infrastructure of the public health system.

Even with all that has happened in recent years in the United States and around the world, the achievement of good health remains a worldwide goal of the twenty-first century. Governments, private organizations, and individuals throughout the world are working to improve health. Although individual actions to improve one's own personal health certainly contribute to the overall health of the community, organized community actions are often necessary when health problems exceed the resources of any one individual. When such actions are not taken, the health of the entire community is at risk.

This chapter introduces the concepts and principles of community health, explains how community health differs from personal health, and provides a brief history of community health. Some of the key health problems facing Americans are also described, and an outlook for the twenty-first century is provided.

BOX 1 A Look Back on the Twentieth Century in the United States

As the twentieth century came to a close, the overall health status and life expectancy in the United States were at all-time highs. Since 1900, the average life span of people in the United States had lengthened by more than 30 years; 25 of these years have been attributed to advances in public health.[2] There were many public health achievements that can be linked to this gain in life expectancy, however. The Centers for Disease Control and Prevention (CDC), the U.S. government agency charged with protecting the public health of the nation, singled out the "Ten Great Public Health Achievements" in the United States between 1900 and 1999. Some of these achievements will be discussed in greater detail in other chapters of this book where they are more relevant to the content being presented. Here is the entire list:[3]

1. *Vaccination.* Vaccines are now available to protect children and adults against 15 life-threatening or debilitating diseases. Rates of all vaccine-preventable diseases are down more than 97% from peak levels before vaccines were available.[4]
2. *Motor vehicle safety.* A number of advances over the years, including safety belts, air bags, safer cars and roads, and enforcement of drunk driving and other laws, have saved many lives.[4]
3. *Safer workplaces.* A number of voluntary and mandatory practices in the workplace have created a much safer work environment. In the early 1900s, the work-related death rate was about 21 per 100,000. By the mid-1990s, that number had dropped to about 4 per 100,000.[5]
4. *Control of infectious diseases.* At the beginning of the twentieth century, the leading causes of death were infectious diseases, but by mid-century many of these diseases were under control. This control can be attributed to cleaner water, improved sanitation, and antibiotics.
5. *Decline of deaths from coronary heart disease and stroke.* Although these remain the leading causes of death, significant progress has been made in reducing the death rates since 1950. This progress can be attributed to the identification and modification of risk factors such as smoking and high blood pressure, and the improved access to early detection and better treatment.
6. *Safer and healthier foods.* Over the twentieth century much of the microbial contamination of food has been significantly reduced, and the nutritional value of foods has been greatly enhanced.
7. *Healthier mothers and babies.* Infant and maternal mortality rates have decreased 90% and 99%, respectively. This can be attributed to advances in hygiene, nutrition, antibiotics, medical technology, and access to health care.
8. *Family planning.* Advances in family planning and contraceptive services have provided for greater health benefits for mothers and babies and have reduced the transmission of several sexually transmitted diseases.
9. *Fluoridation of drinking water.* Though fluoridation of water only began in the mid-twentieth century, it has played an important role in the reduction of both tooth decay and tooth loss.
10. *Recognition of tobacco use as a health hazard.* Recognition of tobacco as the single most preventable cause of death in the United States has saved the lives and suffering of millions of people in this country.

Definitions

The word *health* means different things to different people. Similarly, there are other words that can be defined in various ways. Some basic terms we will use in this book are defined in the following paragraphs.

Health

The word *health* is derived from *hal,* which means "hale, sound, whole." When it comes to the health of people, the word *health* has been defined in a number of different ways—often in its social context, as when a parent describes the health of a child or when an avid fan defines the health of a professional athlete. The most widely quoted definition of health was the one created by the World Health Organization (WHO) in 1946. That definition states that

health
a dynamic state or condition of the human organism that is multidimensional in nature, a resource for living, and results from a person's interactions with and adaptations to his or her environment; therefore, it can exist in varying degrees and is specific to each individual and his or her situation

"health is a state of complete physical, mental, and social well-being and not merely the absence of disease and infirmity."[6] Further, the WHO has indicated that "health is a resource for everyday life, not the object of living, and is a positive concept emphasizing social and personal resources as well as physical capabilities."[6] Others have stated that health cannot be defined as a state because it is ever changing. Therefore, we have chosen to define **health** as a *dynamic* state or condition of the human organism that is multidimensional (i.e., physical, emotional, social, intellectual, spiritual, and occupational) in nature, a resource for living, and results from a person's interactions with and adaptations to his or her environment. Therefore, it can exist in varying degrees and is specific to each individual and his or her situation. "For example, a person can be healthy while dying, or a person who is a quadriplegic can be healthy in the sense that his or her mental and social well-being are high and physical health is as good as it can be."[7]

A person's health status is dynamic in part because of the many different factors that determine one's health. It is widely accepted that health status is determined by the interaction of five domains: gestational endowments (i.e., genetic makeup), social circumstances (e.g., education, employment, income, poverty, housing, crime, and social cohesion), environmental conditions where people live and work (i.e., toxic agents, microbial agents, and structural hazards), behavioral choices (e.g., diet, physical activity, substance use and abuse), and the availability of quality medical care.[8] "Ultimately, the health fate of each of us is determined by factors acting not mostly in isolation but by our experience where domains interconnect. Whether a gene is expressed can be determined by environmental exposures or behavioral patterns. The nature and consequences of behavioral choices are affected by social circumstances. Our genetic predispositions affect the health care we need, and our social circumstances affect the health care we receive."[9]

Community

community
a group of people who have common characteristics; communities can be defined by location, race, ethnicity, age, occupation, interest in particular problems or outcomes, or other common bonds

Traditionally, a community has been thought of as a geographic area with specific boundaries—for example, a neighborhood, city, county, or state. However, in the context of community health, a **community** is "a group of people who have common characteristics; communities can be defined by location, race, ethnicity, age, occupation, interest in particular problems or outcomes, or common bonds."[10] Today we can even talk about a cyber community.[11] Communities are characterized by the following elements:

> (1) membership—a sense of identity and belonging; (2) common symbol systems—similar language, rituals, and ceremonies; (3) shared values and norms; (4) mutual influence—community members have influence and are influenced by each other; (5) shared needs and commitment to meeting them; and (6) shared emotional connection—members share common history, experiences, and mutual support.[12]

Examples of communities include the people of the city of Columbus (location), the Asian community of San Francisco (race), the Hispanic community of Miami (ethnicity), seniors in the church (age), the business or the banking communities (occupation), the homeless of Indiana (specific problem), those on welfare in Ohio (particular outcome), local union members (common bond), or those who are members of a social network (cyber). A community may be as small as the group of people who live on a residence hall floor at a university or as large as all of the individuals who make up a nation. "A healthy community is a place where people provide leadership in assessing their own resources and needs, where public health and social infrastructure and policies support health, and where essential public health services, including quality health care, are available."[13]

Public, Community, Population, and Global Health

Prior to defining the four terms *public health*, *community health*, *population health*, and *global health*, it is important to note that often the terms are used interchangeably by both laypeople and professionals who work in the various health fields. When the terms are used interchangeably, most people are referring to the collective health of those in society and the actions or activities taken to obtain and maintain that health. The definitions provided here for the four terms more precisely define the group of people in question and the origin of the actions or activities.

Of the four terms, *public health* is the most inclusive. The Institute of Medicine (IOM) defined **public health** in 1988 in its landmark report *The Future of Public Health* as "what we as a society do collectively to assure the conditions in which people can be healthy."[14] The **public health system**, which has been defined as "activities undertaken within the formal structure of government and the associated efforts of private and voluntary organizations and individuals,"[14] is the organizational mechanism for providing such conditions. Even with these formal definitions, some still see public health activities as only those efforts that originate in federal, state, and local governmental public health agencies such as the Centers for Disease Control and Prevention and local (i.e., city and county) health departments.

Community health refers to the health status of a defined group of people and the actions and conditions to promote, protect, and preserve their health. For example, the health status of the people of Muncie, Indiana, and the private and public actions taken to promote, protect, and preserve the health of these people would constitute community health.

The term *population health* is similar to *community health*. The primary difference between these two terms is the degree of organization or identity of the people. **Population health** refers to the health status of people who are not organized and have no identity as a group or locality and the actions and conditions to promote, protect, and preserve their health. Men younger than 50, adolescents, prisoners, and white-collar workers are all examples of populations.[15]

A term that has been used increasingly more in recent years is *global health*. The term "does not have one uniform definition. Several organizations have defined the term, and they generally use it in three different ways: (1) as a state or condition; (2) as a goal; and (3) as a field of study, research, and practice."[16] For our discussion here, and to keep it parallel with the terms we have already defined, we use a definition that defines it as a state or condition. Thus, **global health** is a term that describes "health problems, issues, and concerns that transcend national boundaries, may be influenced by circumstances or experiences in other countries, and are best addressed by cooperative actions and solutions."[17] Therefore, an issue such as the 2009 H1N1 flu pandemic can be viewed as a global health issue. Much of the rise in concern about global health problems comes from the speed of international travel and how easy it is for people who may be infected with a disease to cross borders into another country.

public health
actions that society takes collectively to ensure that the conditions in which people can be healthy can occur

public health system
the organizational mechanism of those activities undertaken within the formal structure of government and the associated efforts of private and voluntary organizations and individuals

community health
the health status of a defined group of people and the actions and conditions to promote, protect, and preserve their health

population health
the health status of people who are not organized and have no identity as a group or locality and the actions and conditions to promote, protect, and preserve their health

global health
describes health problems, issues, and concerns that transcend national boundaries, may be influenced by circumstances or experiences in other countries, and are best addressed by cooperative actions and solutions

Personal Health versus Community Health

To further clarify the definitions presented in this chapter, it is important to distinguish between the terms *personal health activities* and *community health activities.*

Personal Health Activities

Personal health activities are individual actions and decision making that affect the health of an individual or his or her immediate family members or friends. These activities may be preventive or curative in nature but seldom directly affect the behavior of others. Choosing to eat wisely, to regularly wear a safety belt, and to visit the physician are all examples of personal health activities.

Community Health Activities

Community health activities are activities that are aimed at protecting or improving the health of a population or community. Maintenance of accurate birth and death records, protection of the food and water supply, and participating in fund drives for voluntary health organizations such as the American Lung Association are examples of community health activities.

Within this book, you are introduced to the many community health activities and to the organizations that are responsible for carrying them out. The following are some of the key topics that are covered in this text:

- Organizations that contribute to community health
- How communities measure health, disease, injury, and death
- Control of communicable and noncommunicable diseases
- How communities organize to solve health problems
- Community health in schools
- Community health needs of people at different stages of life
- Community health needs of special populations
- Community mental health
- Abuse of alcohol, tobacco, and other drugs
- The health care delivery system
- Environmental health problems
- Intentional and unintentional injuries
- Occupational safety and health

Factors That Affect the Health of a Community

There are a great many factors that affect the health of a community. As a result, the health status of each community is different. These factors may be physical, social, and/or cultural. They also include the ability of the community to organize and work together as a whole as well as the individual behaviors of those in the community (see Figure 1).

FIGURE 1
Factors that affect the health of a community.

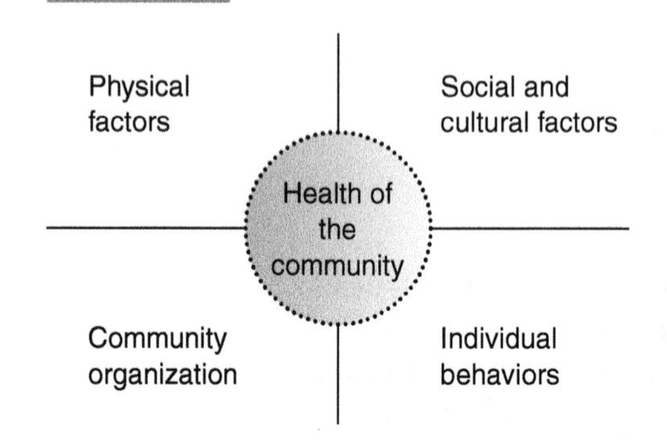

Physical Factors

Physical factors include the influences of geography, the environment, community size, and industrial development.

Geography

A community's health problems can be directly influenced by its altitude, latitude, and climate. In tropical countries where warm, humid temperatures and rain prevail throughout the year, parasitic and infectious diseases are a leading community health problem (see Figure 2). In many tropical countries, survival from these diseases is made more difficult because poor soil conditions result in inadequate food production and malnutrition. In temperate climates with fewer parasitic and infectious diseases and a more than adequate food supply, obesity and heart disease are important community health problems.

Environment

The quality of our environment is directly related to the quality of our stewardship of it. Many experts believe that if we continue to allow uncontrolled population growth and continue to deplete nonrenewable natural resources, succeeding generations will inhabit communities that are less desirable than ours. Many feel that we must accept responsibility for this stewardship and drastically reduce the rate at which we foul the soil, water, and air.

Community Size

The larger the community, the greater its range of health problems and the greater its number of health resources. For example, larger communities have more health professionals and better health facilities than smaller communities. These resources are often needed because communicable diseases can spread more quickly and environmental problems are often more severe in densely populated areas. For example, the amount of trash generated by the approximately 8.3 million people in New York City is many times greater than that generated by the entire state of Wyoming, with its population of about 544,270.

It is important to note that a community's size can have both a positive and negative impact on that community's health. The ability of a community to effectively plan, organize, and utilize its resources can determine whether its size can be used to good advantage.

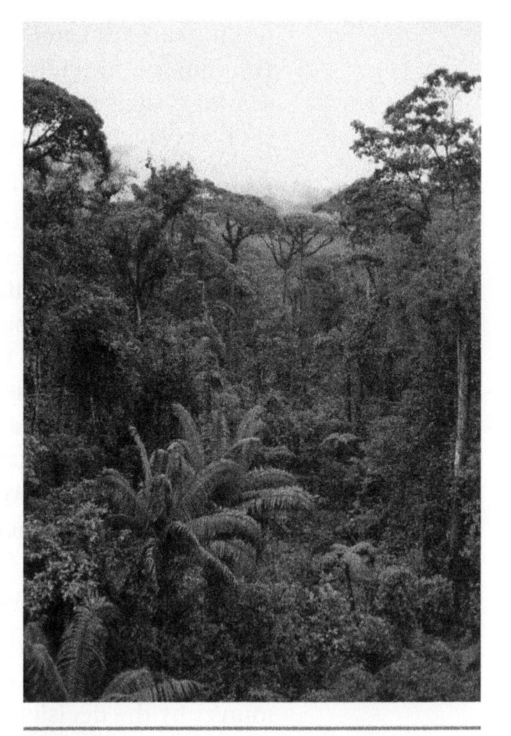

FIGURE 2
In tropical countries, parasitic and infectious diseases are leading community health problems.

Industrial Development

Industrial development, like size, can have either positive or negative effects on the health status of a community. Industrial development provides a community with added resources for community health programs, but it may bring with it environmental pollution and occupational injuries and illnesses. Communities that experience rapid industrial development must eventually regulate the way in which industries (1) obtain raw materials, (2) discharge by-products, (3) dispose of wastes, (4) treat and protect their employees, and (5) clean up environmental accidents. Unfortunately, many of these laws are usually passed only after these communities have suffered significant reductions in the quality of their life and health.

Social and Cultural Factors

Social factors are those that arise from the interaction of individuals or groups within the community. For example, people who live in urban communities, where life is fast-paced, experience higher rates of stress-related illnesses than those who live in rural communities, where life is more leisurely. On the other hand, those in rural areas may not have access to the same quality or selection of health care (i.e., hospitals or medical specialists) that is available to those who live in urban communities.

Cultural factors arise from guidelines (both explicit and implicit) that individuals "inherit" from being a part of a particular society. Culture "teaches us what to fear, what to respect, what to value, and what to regard as relevant in our lives."[18] Some of the factors that contribute to culture are discussed in the following sections.

Beliefs, Traditions, and Prejudices

The beliefs, traditions, and prejudices of community members can affect the health of the community. The beliefs of those in a community about such specific health behaviors as exercise and smoking can influence policy makers on whether or not they will spend money on bike trails and work toward no-smoking ordinances. The traditions of specific ethnic groups can influence the types of food, restaurants, retail outlets, and services available in a community. Prejudices of one specific ethnic or racial group against another can result in acts of violence and crime. Racial and ethnic disparities will continue to put certain groups, such as black Americans or certain religious groups, at greater risk.

Economy

Both national and local economies can affect the health of a community through reductions in health and social services. An economic downturn means lower tax revenues (fewer tax dollars) and fewer contributions to charitable groups. Such actions will result in fewer dollars being available for programs such as welfare, food stamps, community health care, and other community services. This occurs because revenue shortfalls cause agencies to experience budget cuts. With less money, these agencies often must alter their eligibility guidelines, thereby restricting aid to only the neediest individuals. Obviously, many people who had been eligible for assistance before the economic downturn become ineligible.

Employers usually find it increasingly difficult to provide health benefits for their employees as their income drops. The unemployed and underemployed face poverty and deteriorating health. Thus, the cumulative effect of an economic downturn significantly affects the health of the community.

Politics

Those who happen to be in political office can improve or jeopardize the health of their community by the decisions they make. In the most general terms, the argument is over greater or lesser governmental participation in health issues. For example, there has been a long-standing discussion in the United States on the extent to which the government should involve itself in health care. Historically, Democrats have been in favor of such action while Republicans have been against it. State and local politicians also influence the health of their communities each time they vote on health-related measures brought before them, such as a no-smoking ordinance.

Religion

A number of religions have taken a position on health care and health behaviors. For example, some religious communities limit the type of medical treatment their members may receive. Some do not permit immunizations; others do not permit their members to be treated by physicians. Still others prohibit certain foods. For example, Kosher dietary regulations permit Jews to eat the meat only of animals that chew cud and have cloven hooves and the flesh only of fish that have both gills and scales, while still others, like the Native American Church of the Morning Star, use peyote, a hallucinogen, as a sacrament.

Some religious communities actively address moral and ethical issues such as abortion, premarital intercourse, and homosexuality. Still other religions teach health-promoting codes of living to their members. Obviously, religion can affect a community's health positively or negatively (see Figure 3).

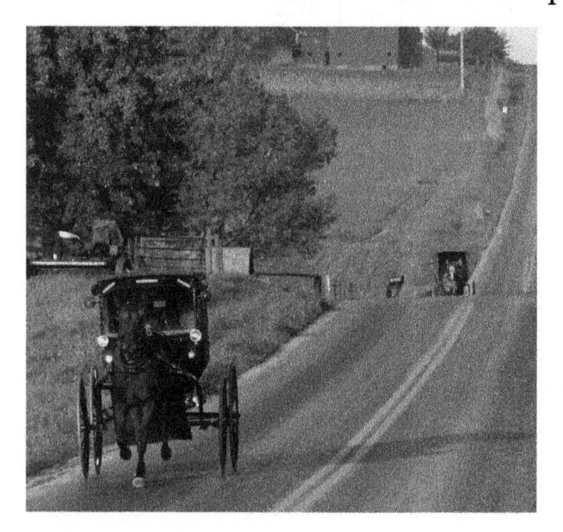

FIGURE 3
Religion can affect a community's health either positively or negatively.

Social Norms

The influence of social norms can be positive or negative and can change over time. Cigarette smoking is a good example. During the 1940s, 1950s, and 1960s, it was socially acceptable to smoke in most settings. As a matter of fact, in 1960, 53% of American men and 32% of American women smoked. Thus, in 1960 it was socially acceptable to be a smoker, especially if you were male. Now, early in the twenty-first century, those percentages have dropped to 23.1% (for males) and 18.3% (for females), and in most public places it has become socially unacceptable to smoke.[19] The lawsuits against tobacco companies by both the state attorneys general and private citizens provide further evidence that smoking has fallen from social acceptability. Because of this change in the social norm, there is less secondhand smoke in many public places, and in turn the health of the community has improved.

Unlike smoking, alcohol consumption represents a continuing negative social norm in America, especially on college campuses. The normal expectation seems to be that drinking is fun (and almost everyone wants to have fun). Despite the fact that most college students are too young to drink legally, approximately 60% of college students drink.[20] It seems fairly obvious that the American alcoholic-beverage industry has influenced our social norms.

Socioeconomic Status

Differences in socioeconomic status, whether "defined by education, employment, or income, both individual- and community-level socioeconomic status have independent effects on health."[21] "In the United States today, the health of poor people is threatened by the adverse environmental conditions of the inner cities, such as lead paint and air pollution, crime, and violence. Poor people also have poorer nutrition, less access to medical care, and more psychological stress."[1] In addition to health care access, higher incomes enable people to afford better housing, live in safer neighborhoods, and increase the opportunity to engage in health-promoting behaviors.[22]

Community Organizing

The way in which a community is able to organize its resources directly influences its ability to intervene and solve problems, including health problems. **Community organizing** "is a process through which communities are helped to identify common problems or goals, mobilize resources, and in other ways develop and implement strategies for reaching their goals they have collectively set."[23] It is not a science but an art of building consensus within a democratic process.[24] If a community can organize its resources effectively into a unified force, it "is likely to produce benefits in the form of increased effectiveness and productivity by reducing duplication of efforts and avoiding the imposition of solutions that are not congruent with the local culture and needs."[13] For example, many communities in the United States have faced community-wide drug problems. Some have been able to organize their resources to reduce or resolve these problems, whereas others have not.

community organizing a process through which communities are helped to identify common problems or goals, mobilize resources, and in other ways develop and implement strategies for reaching their goals they have collectively set

Individual Behavior

The behavior of the individual community members contributes to the health of the entire community. It takes the concerted effort of many—if not most—of the individuals in a community to make a program work. For example, if each individual consciously recycles his or her trash each week, community recycling will be successful. Likewise, if each occupant would wear a safety belt, there could be a significant reduction in the number of facial injuries and deaths from car crashes for the entire community. In another example, the more individuals who become immunized against a specific disease, the slower the disease will spread and the fewer people will be exposed. This concept is known as **herd immunity**.

herd immunity the resistance of a population to the spread of an infectious agent based on the immunity of a high proportion of individuals

A Brief History of Community and Public Health

The history of community and public health is almost as long as the history of civilization. This brief summary provides an account of some of the accomplishments and failures in

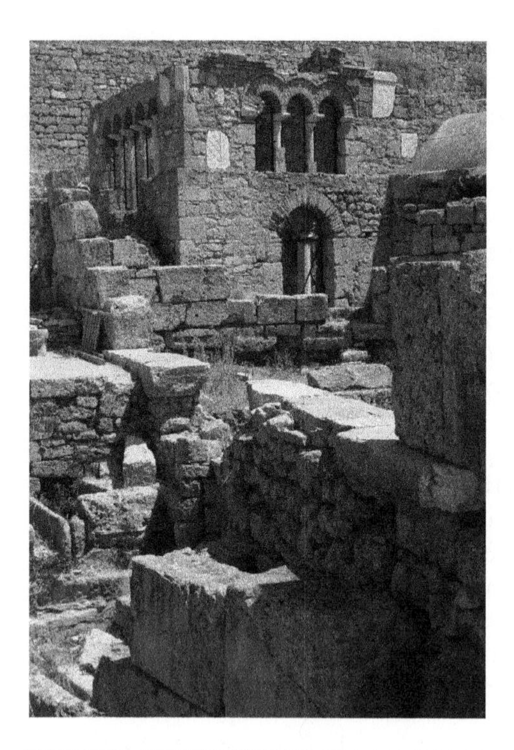

FIGURE 4
Archeological findings reveal community health practices of the past.

community and public health. It is hoped that a knowledge of the past will enable us to better prepare for future challenges to our community's health.

Earliest Civilizations

In all likelihood, the earliest community health practices went unrecorded. Perhaps these practices involved taboos against defecation within the tribal communal area or near the source of drinking water. Perhaps they involved rites associated with burial of the dead. Certainly, the use of herbs for the prevention and curing of diseases and communal assistance with childbirth are practices that predate archeological records.

Excavations at sites of some of the earliest known civilizations, dating from about 2000 B.C., have uncovered archeological evidence of community health activities (see Figure 4). A combination of additional archeological findings and written history provides much more evidence of community health activities through the seventeenth century. Box 2 provides a timeline and some of the highlights of that history for the Ancient Societies (before 500 B.C.), the Classical Cultures (500 B.C.–A.D. 500), the Middle Ages (A.D. 500–1500), and the period of Renaissance and Exploration (1500–1700)

The Eighteenth Century

The eighteenth century was characterized by industrial growth. Despite the beginnings of recognition of the nature of disease, living conditions were hardly conducive to good health. Cities were overcrowded, and water supplies were inadequate and often unsanitary. Streets were usually unpaved, filthy, and heaped with trash and garbage. Many homes had unsanitary dirt floors.

Workplaces were unsafe and unhealthy. A substantial portion of the workforce was made up of the poor, which included children, who were forced to work long hours as indentured servants. Many of these jobs were unsafe or involved working in unhealthy environments, such as textile factories and coal mines.

One medical advance made at the end of the eighteenth century deserves mention because of its significance for public health. In 1796, Dr. Edward Jenner successfully demonstrated the process of vaccination as a protection against smallpox. He did this by inoculating a boy with material from a cowpox (*Vaccinia*) pustule. When challenged later with material from a smallpox (*Variola*) pustule, the boy remained healthy.

Dr. Jenner's discovery remains as one of the great discoveries of all time for both medicine and for public health. Prior to Dr. Jenner's discovery, millions died or were severely disfigured by smallpox (see Figure 5). The only known prevention had been "variolation," inoculation with smallpox material itself. This was a risky procedure because people sometimes became quite ill with smallpox. Nonetheless, during the American Revolution, General George Washington ordered the Army of the American Colonies "variolated." He did this so that he could be sure an epidemic of smallpox would not wipe out his colonial forces.[27] Interestingly enough, the average age at death for one living in the United States during this time was 29 years.

Following the American Revolution, George Washington ordered the first U.S. census for the purpose of the apportionment of representation in the House of Representatives. The

BOX 2

Timeline and Highlights of Community and Public Health Prior to 1700

A. Early Civilizations
   1. Ancient Societies (before 500 B.C.)
      a. Prior to 2000 B.C.: Archeological findings provide evidence of sewage disposal and written medical prescriptions.
      b. Circa 1900 B.C.: Perhaps the earliest written record of public health was the Code of Hammurabi; included laws for physicians and health practices.[25]
      c. Circa 1500 B.C.: Bible's Book of Leviticus written; includes guidelines for personal cleanliness and sanitation.[25]
   2. Classical Cultures (500 B.C.–A.D. 500)
      a. Fifth and sixth centuries B.C.: Evidence that Greek men participated in games of strength and skill and swam in public facilities.[26]
      b. Greeks were involved in practice of community sanitation; involved in obtaining water from sources far away and not just local wells.[27]
      c. Romans were community minded; improved on community sanitation of Greeks; built aqueducts to transport water from miles away; built sewer systems; created regulation for building construction, refuse removal, and street cleaning and repair;[25] created hospitals as infirmaries for slaves.[28]
      d. Christians created hospitals as benevolent charitable organizations.[28]
      e. A.D. 476: Roman Empire fell and most public health activities ceased.

B. Middle Ages (A.D. 500–1500)
   a. A.D. 500–1000 (Dark Ages): Growing revulsion for Roman materialism and a growth of spirituality; health problems were considered to have both spiritual causes and spiritual solutions;[28] time referred to as the **spiritual era of public health**.
   b. Failure to take into account the role of the physical and biological environment in the causation of communicable diseases resulted in many unrelenting epidemics in which millions suffered and died.
      - Deadliest epidemics were from plague ("black death"); occurred in A.D. 543 and 1348 (this one killed 25 million; half of population of London lost and in some parts of France only 1 in 10 survived).[25]
      - A.D. 1200: More than 19,000 leper houses.
      - Other epidemics of period: Smallpox, diphtheria, measles, influenza, tuberculosis, anthrax, and trachoma.
      - A.D. 1492: Syphilis epidemic was last epidemic of the period.

C. Renaissance and Exploration (1500–1700)
   a. Rebirth of thinking about the nature of world and humankind.
   b. Belief that disease was caused by environmental, not spiritual, factors; for example, the term *malaria*, meaning bad air, is a direct reference to humid or swampy air.
   c. Observation of ill led to more accurate descriptions of symptoms and outcomes of diseases; observations led to first recognition of whooping cough, typhus, scarlet fever, and malaria as distinct and separate diseases.[27]
   d. Epidemics (e.g., smallpox, malaria, and plague) still rampant; plague epidemic killed 68,596 (15% of the population) in London in 1665.
   e. Explorers, conquerors, and merchants and their crews spread disease to colonists and indigenous people throughout the New World.

census, first taken in 1790, is still conducted every 10 years and serves as an invaluable source of information for community health planning.

As the eighteenth century came to a close, a young United States faced numerous disease problems, including continuing outbreaks of smallpox, cholera, typhoid fever, and yellow fever. Yellow fever outbreaks usually occurred in port cities such as Charleston, Baltimore, New York, and New Orleans, where ships arrived to dock from tropical America. The greatest single epidemic of yellow fever in America occurred in Philadelphia in 1793, where there were an estimated 23,000 cases, including 4,044 deaths in a population estimated at only 37,000.[29]

In response to these continuing epidemics and the need to address other mounting health problems, such as sanitation and protection of the water supply, several governmental

spiritual era of public health
a time during the Middle Ages when the causation of communicable disease was linked to spiritual forces

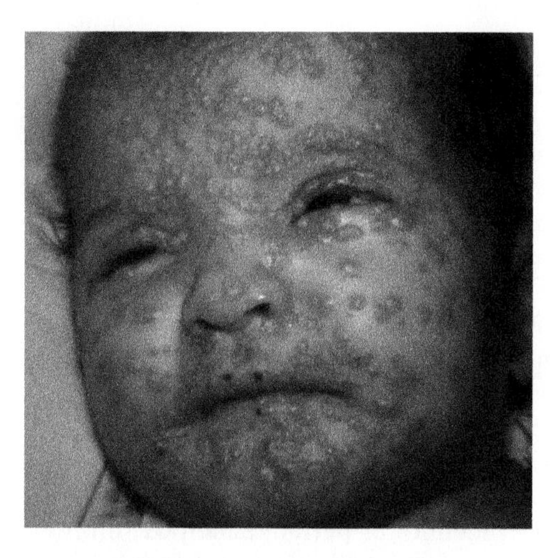

FIGURE 5
Prior to the elimination of smallpox, millions died or were severely disfigured by the disease.

health agencies were created. In 1798, the Marine Hospital Service (forerunner to the U.S. Public Health Service) was formed to deal with disease that was occurring onboard water vessels. By 1799, several of America's largest cities, including Boston, Philadelphia, New York, and Baltimore, also had founded municipal boards of health.

The Nineteenth Century

During the first half of the nineteenth century, few remarkable advancements in public health occurred. Living conditions in Europe and England remained unsanitary, and industrialization led to an even greater concentration of the population within cities. However, better agricultural methods led to improved nutrition for many.

During this period, America enjoyed westward expansion, characterized by a spirit of pioneering, self-sufficiency, and rugged individualism. The federal government's approach to health problems was characterized by the French term *laissez faire,* meaning noninterference. There were also few health regulations or health departments in rural areas. Health quackery thrived; this was truly a period when "buyer beware" was good advice.

Epidemics continued in major cities in both Europe and America. In 1854, another cholera epidemic struck London. Dr. John Snow studied the epidemic and hypothesized that the disease was being caused by the drinking water from the Broad Street pump. He obtained permission to remove the pump handle, and the epidemic was abated (see Figure 6). Snow's action was remarkable because it predated the discovery that microorganisms can cause disease. The predominant theory of contagious disease at the time was the "miasmas theory." According to this theory, vapors, or miasmas, were the source of many diseases. The miasmas theory remained popular throughout much of the nineteenth century.

In the United States in 1850, Lemuel Shattuck drew up a health report for the Commonwealth of Massachusetts that outlined the public health needs for the state. It included recommendations for the establishment of boards of health, the collection of vital statistics, the implementation of sanitary measures, and research on diseases. Shattuck also recommended health education and controlling exposure to alcohol, smoke, adulterated food, and nostrums (quack medicines).[25] Although some of his recommendations took years to implement (the Massachusetts Board of Health was not founded until 1869), the significance of Shattuck's report is such that 1850 is a key date in American public health; it marks the beginning of the **modern era of public health**.

modern era of public health
the era of public health that began in 1850 and continues today

Real progress in the understanding of the causes of many communicable diseases occurred during the last quarter of the nineteenth century. One of the obstacles to progress was the theory of spontaneous generation, the idea that living organisms could arise from inorganic or nonliving matter. Akin to this idea was the thought that one type of contagious microbe could change into another type of organism.

In 1862, Louis Pasteur of France proposed his germ theory of disease. Throughout the 1860s and 1870s, he and others carried out experiments and made observations that supported this theory and disproved spontaneous generation. Pasteur is generally given credit for providing the death blow to the theory of spontaneous generation.

It was the German scientist Robert Koch who developed the criteria and procedures necessary to establish that a particular microbe, and no other, causes a particular disease. His first demonstration, with the anthrax bacillus, was in 1876. Between 1877 and the end of the century, the identity of numerous bacterial disease agents was established, including those that caused gonorrhea, typhoid fever, leprosy, tuberculosis, cholera, diphtheria, tetanus, pneumonia, plague, and dysentery. This period (1875-1900) has come to be known as the **bacteriological period of public health**.

Although most scientific discoveries in the late nineteenth century were made in Europe, there were significant public health achievements occurring in America as well. The first law prohibiting the adulteration of milk was passed in 1856, the first sanitary survey was carried out in New York City in 1864, and the American Public Health Association was founded in 1872. The Marine Hospital Service gained new powers of inspection and investigation under the Port Quarantine Act of 1878.[25] In 1890, the pasteurization of milk was introduced, and in 1891 meat inspection began. It was also during this time that nurses were first hired by industries (in 1895) and schools (in 1899). Also in 1895, septic tanks were introduced for sewage treatment. In 1900, Major Walter Reed of the U.S. Army announced that yellow fever was transmitted by mosquitoes.

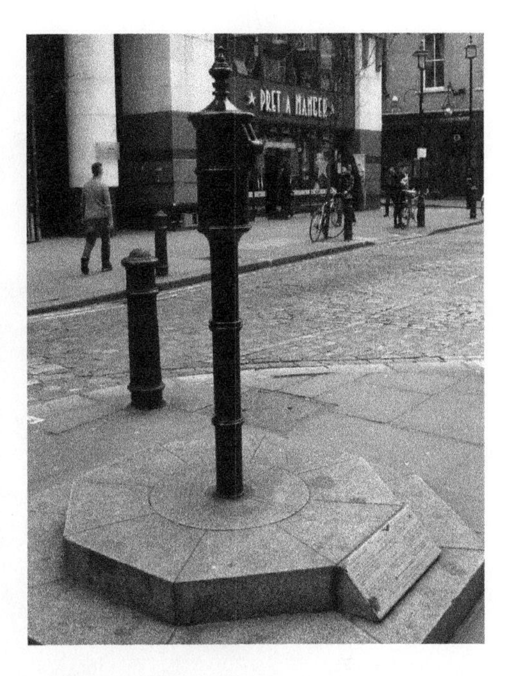

FIGURE 6

In London, England, 1854, John Snow helped interrupt a cholera epidemic by having the handle removed from this pump, located on Broad Street.

The Twentieth Century

As the twentieth century began, life expectancy was still less than 50 years.[30] The leading causes of death were communicable diseases—influenza, pneumonia, tuberculosis, and infections of the gastrointestinal tract. Other communicable diseases, such as typhoid fever, malaria, and diphtheria, also killed many people.

There were other health problems as well. Thousands of children were afflicted with conditions characterized by noninfectious diarrhea or by bone deformity. Although the symptoms of pellagra and rickets were known and described, the causes of these ailments remained a mystery at the turn of the century. Discovery that these conditions resulted from vitamin deficiencies was slow because some scientists were searching for bacterial causes.

bacteriological period of public health
the period of 1875–1900, during which the causes of many bacterial diseases were discovered

Vitamin deficiency diseases and one of their contributing conditions, poor dental health, were extremely common in the slum districts of both European and American cities. The unavailability of adequate prenatal and postnatal care meant that deaths associated with pregnancy and childbirth were also high.

Health Resources Development Period (1900–1960)

Much growth and development took place during the 60-year period from 1900 to 1960. Because of the growth of health care facilities and providers, this period of time is referred to as the **health resources development period**. This period can be further divided into the reform phase (1900-1920), the 1920s, the Great Depression and World War II, and the postwar years.

health resources development period
the years of 1900–1960, a time of great growth in health care facilities and providers

The Reform Phase (1900-1920)

By the beginning of the twentieth century, there was a growing concern about the many social problems in America. The remarkable discoveries in microbiology made in the previous years had not dramatically improved the health of the average citizen. By 1910, the urban population had grown to 45% of the total population (up from 19% in 1860). Much of the growth was the result of immigrants who came to America for the jobs created by new industries (see Figure 7). Northern cities were also swelling from the northward migration of black Americans from the southern states. Many of these workers had to accept poorly

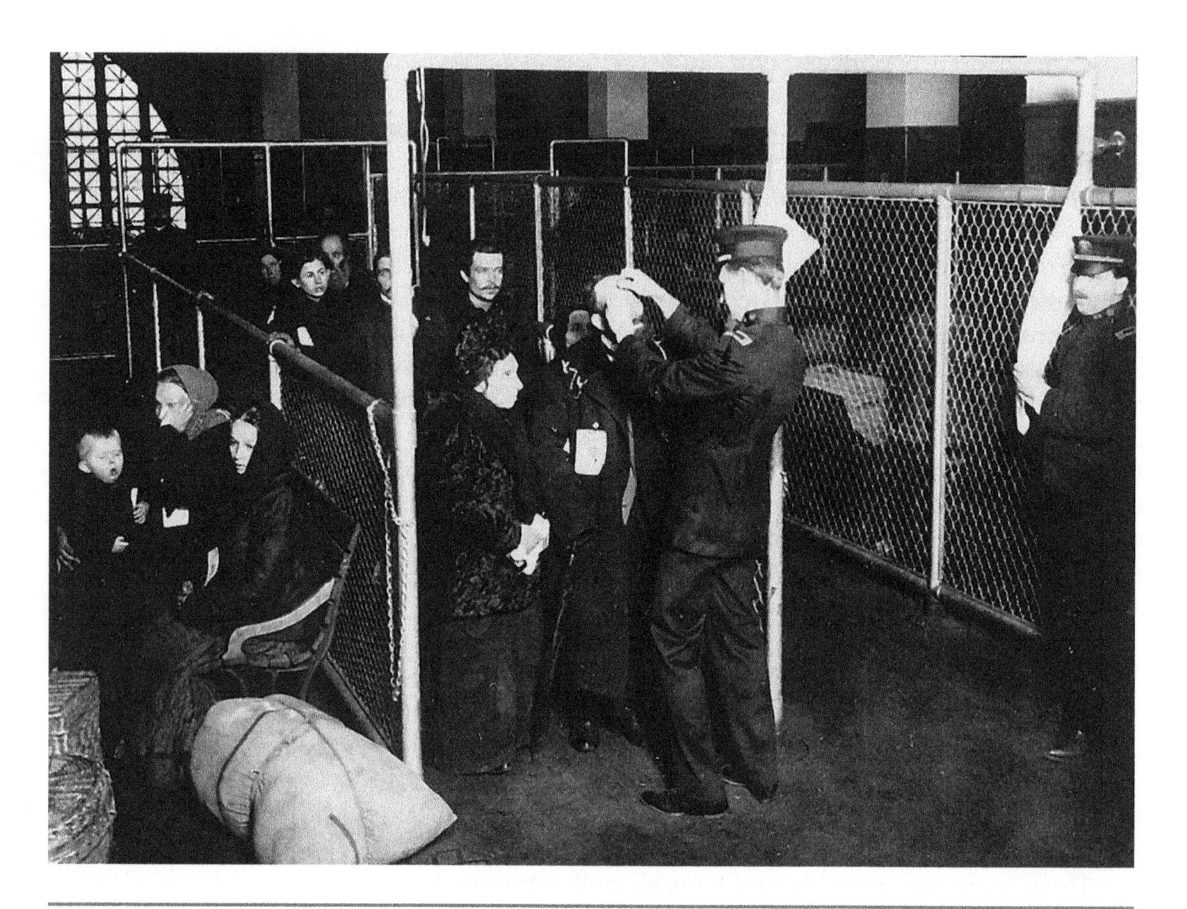

FIGURE 7
Ellis Island immigration between 1860 and 1910 resulted in dramatic increases in the urban population in America.

paying jobs involving hard labor and low wages. There was also a deepening chasm between the upper and lower classes, and social critics began to clamor for reform.

reform phase of public health the years of 1900–1920, characterized by social movements to improve health conditions in cities and in the workplace

The years 1900 to 1920 have been called the **reform phase of public health**. The plight of the immigrants working in the meat packing industry was graphically depicted by Upton Sinclair in his book *The Jungle*. Sinclair's goal was to draw attention to unsafe working conditions. What he achieved was greater governmental regulation of the food industry through the passage of the Pure Food and Drugs Act of 1906.

The reform movement was broad, involving both social and moral as well as health issues. Edward T. Devine noted in 1909 that "Ill health is perhaps the most constant of the attendants of poverty."[30] The reform movement finally took hold when it became evident to the majority that neither the discoveries of the causes of many communicable diseases nor the continuing advancement of industrial production could overcome continuing disease and poverty. Even by 1917, the United States ranked fourteenth of 16 "progressive" nations in maternal death rate.[30]

Although the relationship between occupation and disease had been pointed out 200 years earlier in Europe, occupational health in America in 1900 was an unknown quantity. However, in 1910 the first International Congress on Occupational Diseases was held in Chicago.[31] That same year, the state of New York passed a tentative Workman's Compensation Act, and over the next 10 years most other states passed similar laws.[22] Also in 1910, the U.S. Bureau of Mines was created and the first clinic for occupational diseases was established in New York at Cornell Medical College.[30] By 1910, the movement for healthier conditions in the workplace was well established.

This period also saw the birth of the first national-level volunteer health agencies. The first of these agencies was the National Association for the Study and Prevention of Tuberculosis, which was formed in 1902. It arose from the first local voluntary health agency, the Pennsylvania Society for the Prevention of Tuberculosis, organized in 1892.[32] The American Cancer Society, Inc., was founded in 1913. That same year, the Rockefeller Foundation was established in New York. This philanthropic foundation has funded a great many public health projects, including work on hookworm and pellagra, and the development of a vaccine against yellow fever.

Another movement that began about this time was that of public health nursing. The first school nursing program was begun in New York City in 1902. In 1918, the first School of Public Health was established at Johns Hopkins University in Baltimore. This was followed by establishment of another school at Harvard University in 1923. Also in 1918 was the birth of school health instruction as we know it today.

These advances were matched with similar advances by governmental bodies. The Marine Hospital Service was renamed the Public Health and Marine Hospital Service in 1902 in keeping with its growing responsibilities. In 1912, it became the U.S. Public Health Service.[25]

By 1900, 38 states had state health departments. The rest followed during the first decades of the twentieth century. The first two local (county) health departments were established in 1911, one in Guilford County, North Carolina, and the other in Yakima County, Washington.

The 1920s

In comparison with the preceding period, the 1920s represented a decade of slow growth in public health, except for a few health projects funded by the Rockefeller and Millbank foundations. Prohibition resulted in a decline in the number of alcoholics and alcohol-related deaths. Although the number of county health departments had risen to 467 by 1929, 77% of the rural population still lived in areas with no health services.[32] However, it was during this period in 1922 that the first professional preparation program for health educators was begun at Columbia University by Thomas D. Wood, MD, whom many consider the father of health education. The life expectancy in 1930 had risen to 59.7 years.

The Great Depression and World War II

Until the Great Depression (1929–1935), individuals and families in need of social and medical services were dependent on friends and relatives, private charities, voluntary agencies, community chests, and churches. By 1933, after 3 years of economic depression, it became evident that private resources could never meet the needs of all the people who needed assistance. The drop in tax revenues during the Depression also reduced health department budgets and caused a virtual halt in the formation of new local health departments.[32]

Beginning in 1933, President Franklin D. Roosevelt created numerous agencies and programs for public works as part of his New Deal. Much of the money was used for public health, including the control of malaria, the building of hospitals and laboratories, and the construction of municipal water and sewer systems.

The Social Security Act of 1935 marked the beginning of the government's major involvement in social issues, including health. This act provided substantial support for state health departments and their programs, such as maternal and child health and sanitary facilities. As progress against the communicable diseases became visible, some turned their attention toward other health problems, such as cancer. The National Cancer Institute was formed in 1937.

America's involvement in World War II resulted in severe restrictions on resources available for public health programs. Immediately following the conclusion of the war, however, many of the medical discoveries made during wartime made their way into civilian medical practice. Two examples are the antibiotic penicillin, used for treating pneumonia, rheumatic fever, syphilis, and strep throat, and the insecticide DDT, used for killing insects that transmit diseases.

During World War II, the Communicable Disease Center was established in Atlanta, Georgia. Now called the Centers for Disease Control and Prevention (CDC), it has become the premier epidemiological center of the world.

The Postwar Years

Following the end of World War II, there was still concern about medical care and the adequacy of the facilities in which that care could be administered. In 1946, Congress passed the National Hospital Survey and Construction Act (the Hill-Burton Act). The goal of the legislation was to improve the distribution of medical care and to enhance the quality of hospitals. From 1946 through the 1960s, hospital construction occurred at a rapid rate with relatively little thought given to planning. Likewise, attempts to set national health priorities or to establish a national health agenda were virtually nonexistent.

The two major health events in the 1950s were the development of a vaccine to prevent polio and President Eisenhower's heart attack. The latter event helped America to focus on its number 1 killer, heart disease. When the president's physician suggested exercise, some Americans heeded his advice and began to exercise on a regular basis.

Period of Social Engineering (1960–1973)

The 1960s marked the beginning of a period when the federal government once again became active in health matters. The primary reason for this involvement was the growing realization that many Americans were still not reaping any of the benefits of 60 years of medical advances. These Americans, most of whom were poor or elderly, either lived in underserved areas or simply could not afford to purchase medical services.

Medicare
government health insurance for older adults and those with certain disabilities

Medicaid
government health insurance for the poor

In 1965, Congress passed the Medicare and Medicaid bills (amendments to the Social Security Act of 1935). **Medicare** assists in the payment of medical bills for older adults and certain people with disabilities, and **Medicaid** assists in the payment of medical bills for the poor. These pieces of legislation helped provide medical care for millions who would not otherwise have received it, and this legislation also improved standards in health care facilities. Unfortunately, the influx of federal dollars accelerated the rate of increase in the cost of health care for everyone. As a result, the 1970s, 1980s, and the 1990s saw repeated attempts and failures to bring the growing costs of health care under control.

Period of Health Promotion (1974–Present)

By the mid-1970s, it had become apparent that the greatest potential for saving lives and reducing health care costs in America was to be achieved through means other than health care.

> Most scholars, policymakers, and practitioners in health promotion would pick 1974 as the turning point that marks the beginning of health promotion as a significant component of national health policy in the twentieth century. That year Canada published its landmark policy statement, *A New Perspective on the Health of Canadians*.[33] In [1976] the United States, Congress passed PL 94-317, the Health Information and Health Promotion Act, which created the Office of Health Information and Health Promotion, later renamed the Office of Disease Prevention and Health Promotion.[34]

In the late 1970s, the Centers for Disease Control conducted a study that examined premature deaths (defined then as deaths prior to age 65, but now as deaths prior to age 75) in the United States in 1977. That study revealed that approximately 48% of all premature deaths could be traced to one's lifestyle or health behavior—choices that people make. Lifestyles characterized by a lack of exercise, unhealthy diets, smoking, uncontrolled hypertension, and the inability to control stress were found to be contributing factors to premature mortality.[35] This led the way for the U.S. government's publication *Healthy People: The*

Surgeon General's Report on Health Promotion and Disease Prevention.[36] "This document brought together much of what was known about the relationship of personal behavior and health status. The document also presented a 'personal responsibility' model that provided Americans with the prescription for reducing their health risks and increasing their chances for good health."[37]

Healthy People was then followed by the release of the first set of health goals and objectives for the nation, called *Promoting Health/Preventing Disease: Objectives for the Nation.*[38] At the time this edition of this book was going to press, the fourth edition of these goals and objectives, *Healthy People 2020*, was about to be released. Since their inception, these *Healthy People* documents have defined the nation's health agenda and guided its health policy since their inception (see Box 3).

BOX 3

TIMELINE AND HIGHLIGHTS OF COMMUNITY AND PUBLIC HEALTH FROM 1700–2000

A. Eighteenth Century (1700s)
   1. Period characterized by industrial growth; workplaces were unsafe and unhealthy
   2. 1790: first U.S. census
   3. 1793: yellow fever epidemic in Philadelphia
   4. 1796: Dr. Edward Jenner successfully demonstrated smallpox vaccination
   5. 1798: Marine Hospital Service (forerunner to U.S. Public Health Service) was formed
   6. By 1799: several of America's largest cities, including Boston, Philadelphia, New York, and Baltimore, had municipal boards of health

B. First Half of Nineteenth Century (1800–1848)
   1. U.S. government's approach to health was laissez faire
   2. 1813: first visiting nurse in United States

C. Second Half of 19th Century (1848-1900)
   1. 1849,1854: London cholera epidemics
   2. 1850: Modern era of public health begins
   3. 1850: Shattuck's report
   4. 1854: Snow has pump handle removed from Broad Street pump
   5. 1863: Pasteur proposed germ theory
   6. 1872: American Public Health Association founded
   7. 1875-1900: Bacteriological period of public health
   8. 1876: Koch established relationship between a particular microbe and a particular disease
   9. 1900: Reed announced that yellow fever was transmitted by mosquitos

D. Twentieth Century
   1. Health Resources Development Period (1900-1960)
      a. The Reform Phase (1900-1920)
         - 1902: First national-level voluntary health agency created
         - 1906: Sinclair's *The Jungle* published
         - 1910: First International Congress on Occupational Diseases
         - 1910: 45% of U.S. population was in the cities
         - 1911: First local health department established
         - 1913: American Cancer Society founded
         - 1917: United States ranked 14th of 16 in maternal death rate
         - 1918: Birth of school health instruction
         - 1918: First school of public health established in United States
   2. 1920s
      a. 1922: Wood created first professional preparation program for health educators
      b. 1930: Life expectancy in the United States was 59.7 years
   3. The Great Depression and WWII
      a. 1933: New Deal; included unsuccessful attempt at national health care program
      b. 1935: Social Security Act passed
      c. 1937: National Cancer Institute formed
   4. Postwar Years
      a. 1946: National Hospital Survey and Construction (Hill-Burton) Act passed
      b. 1952: Development of polio vaccine
      c. 1955: Eisenhower's heart attack

E. Period of Social Engineering (1960-1973)
   1. 1965: Medicare and Medicaid bills passed

F. Period of Health Promotion (1974-present)
   1. 1974: Nixon's unsuccessful attempt at national health care program
   2. 1974: *A New Perspective on the Health of Canadians* published
   3. 1976: Health Information and Health Promotion Act passed
   4. 1979: *Healthy People* published
   5. 1980: *Promoting Health/Preventing Disease: Objectives of the Nation* published
   6. 1990: *Healthy People 2000* published
   7. 1997: Clinton's unsuccessful attempt at a national health care program
   8. 2000: *Healthy People 2010* published

Community Health in the Early 2000s

Early in the new millennium, it is widely agreed that although decisions about health are an individual's responsibility to a significant degree, society has an obligation to provide an environment in which the achievement of good health is possible and encouraged. Furthermore, many recognize that certain segments of our population whose disease and death rates exceed the general population may require additional resources, including education, to achieve good health.

The American people face a number of serious public health problems. These problems include the continuing rise in health care costs, growing environmental concerns, the ever-present lifestyle diseases, emerging and reemerging communicable diseases, serious substance abuse problems, and disasters, both natural and humanmade. In the paragraphs that follow, we have elaborated on each of these problems briefly because they seem to represent a significant portion of the community health agenda for the years ahead.

Health Care Delivery

In the previous edition of this book, in this section we wrote about the large number of Americans who were uninsured and the rising cost of health care and how these problems had detrimental effects on both the physical health of individuals and the economic health of the nation. In March 2010, significant changes were made to the U.S. health care system when President Barack Obama signed the Affordable Care Act (ACA) into law. Though the law has many components, the primary focus is to increase the number of Americans with health insurance.

The ACA does this, but by providing health insurance to an additional 32 million Americans, the costs will also go up, which will continue to make U.S. health care the most expensive in the world. In 2010, health expenditures were projected to be almost $2.6 trillion, consume 17.3% of the gross domestic product (GDP), and are expected to reach $4.5 trillion and 19.3% of the GDP by 2019.[39] America spends more per capita annually on health care (estimated at $8,290 in 2010)[39] than any other nation. The cost of health care is an issue that still needs to be addressed.

Environmental Problems

Millions of Americans live in communities where the air is unsafe to breathe, the water is unsafe to drink, or solid waste is disposed of improperly. With a few minor exceptions, the rate at which we pollute our environment continues to increase. Many Americans still believe that our natural resources are unlimited and that their individual contributions to the overall pollution are insignificant. In actuality, we must improve on our efforts in resource preservation and energy conservation if our children are to enjoy an environment as clean as ours. These environmental problems are compounded by the fact that the world population continues to grow; it is now more than 6.9 billion people and expected to reach 8 billion by the year 2026.[40]

Lifestyle Diseases

The leading causes of death in the United States today are not the communicable diseases that were so feared 100 years ago but chronic illnesses resulting from unwise lifestyle choices. The prevalence of obesity and diseases like diabetes is increasing. The four leading causes of death in the early 2000s are heart disease, cancer, chronic lower respiratory diseases, and stroke.[41] Although it is true that everyone has to die from some cause sometime, too many Americans die prematurely because of their unhealthy lifestyles. In the latter part of the twentieth century, it was known that better control of behavioral risk factors alone—such as lack of exercise, poor diet, use of tobacco and drugs, and alcohol abuse—could prevent between 40% and 70% of all premature deaths, one-third of all acute disabilities, and

Table 1
Comparison of Most Common Causes of Death and Actual Causes of Death

Most Common Causes of Death, United States, 2008	Actual Causes of Death, United States, 2000
1. Diseases of the heart	1. Tobacco
2. Malignant neoplasms (cancers)	2. Poor diet and physical inactivity
3. Chronic lower respiratory diseases	3. Alcohol consumption
4. Cerebrovascular diseases (stroke)	4. Microbial agents
5. Unintentional injuries (accidents)	5. Toxic agents
7. Alzheimer's disease	6. Motor vehicles
6. Diabetes mellitus	7. Firearms
8. Influenza and pneumonia	8. Sexual behavior
9. Nephritis, nephrotic syndrome, and nephrosis	9. Illicit drug use
10. Septicemia	

Sources: Miniño, A. M., J. Q. Xu, and K. D. Kochanek (2010). "Deaths: Preliminary Data for 2008." *National Vital Statistics Reports*, 59(2): Hyattsville, MD: National Center for Health Statistics; Mokdad, A. H., J. S. Marks, D. F. Stroup, and J. L. Gerberding (2004). "Actual Causes of Death, in the United States, 2000." *Journal of the American Medical Association*, 291(10): 1238–1245; and Mokdad, A. H., J. S. Marks, D. F. Stroup, and J. L. Gerberding (2005). "Correction: Actual Causes of Death, in the United States, 2000." *Journal of the American Medical Association*, 293(3): 293–294.

two-thirds of chronic disabilities.[42] Now into the twenty-first century, behavior patterns continue to "represent the single most prominent domain of influence over health prospects in the United States."[9] (See Table 1.)

Communicable Diseases

Although communicable (infectious) diseases no longer constitute the leading causes of death in the United States, they remain a concern for several reasons. First, they are the primary reason for days missed at school or at work. The success in reducing the life-threatening nature of these diseases has made many Americans complacent about obtaining vaccinations or taking other precautions against contracting these diseases. With the exception of smallpox, none of these diseases has been eradicated, although several should have been, such as measles.

Second, as new communicable diseases continue to appear, old ones such as tuberculosis reemerge, sometimes in drug-resistant forms, demonstrating that communicable diseases still represent a serious community health problem in America. Legionnaires' disease, toxic shock syndrome, Lyme disease, acquired immunodeficiency syndrome (AIDS), and severe acute respiratory syndrome (SARS) are diseases that were unknown only 30 years ago. The first cases of AIDS were reported in June 1981.[43] By August 1989, 100,000 cases had been reported,[44] and it took only an additional two years to report the second 100,000 cases.[45] By 2006, more than a million cases of the disease had been reported to the CDC.[46] (See Figure 8.) The total number of cases continues to grow with close to 40,000 new cases being diagnosed each year.[47] Also, diseases that were once only found in animals are now crossing over to human populations and causing much concern and action. Included in

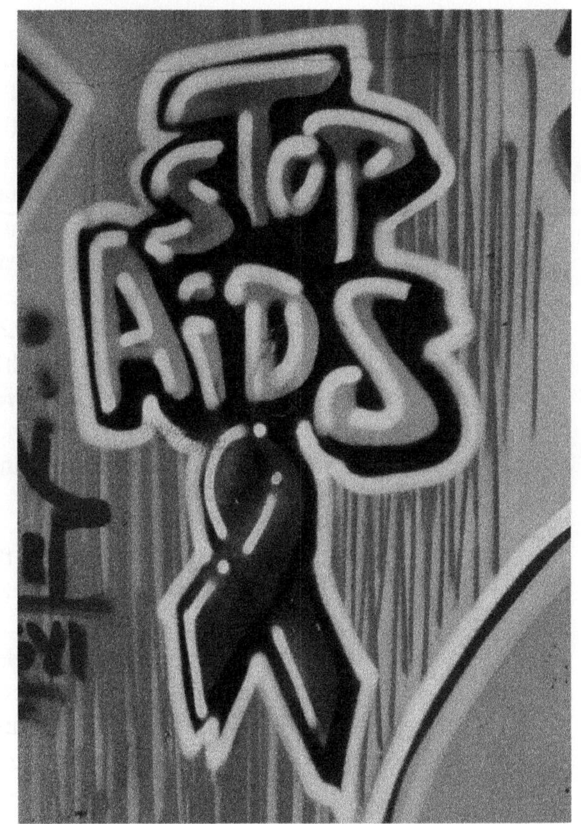

FIGURE 8
AIDS is one of the most feared communicable diseases today.

this group of diseases are avian flu, *Escherichia coli* O157:H7, hantavirus, mad cow disease, and SARS.[1]

bioterrorism
the threatened or intentional release of biological agents for the purpose of influencing the conduct of government or intimidating or coercing a civilian population to further political or social objectives

Third, and maybe the most disturbing, is the use of communicable diseases for bioterrorism. **Bioterrorism** involves "the threatened or intentional release of biological agents (virus, bacteria, or their toxins) for the purpose of influencing the conduct of government or intimidating or coercing a civilian population to further political or social objectives. These agents can be released by way of the air (as aerosols) food, water or insects."[10] Concern in the United States over bioterrorism was heightened after 9/11 and the subsequent intentional distribution of *Bacillus anthracis* spores through the U.S. postal system (the anthrax mailings). The anthrax mailings resulted in 22 people developing anthrax, 5 of whom died. In addition, thousands more were psychologically affected, and between 10 thousand and 20 thousand people were advised to take postexposure prophylactic treatment because they were at known or potential risk for inhalational anthrax.[48]

Alcohol and Other Drug Abuse

"Abuse of legal and illegal drugs has become a national problem that costs this country thousands of lives and billions of dollars each year. Alcohol and other drugs are often associated with unintentional injuries, domestic violence, and violent crimes."[49] Federal, state, and local governments as well as private agencies attempt to address the supply and demand problems associated with the abuse of alcohol and other drugs, but a significant challenge remains for America.

Health Disparities

health disparities
the difference in health among different populations

It has long been "recognized that some individuals are healthier than others and that some live longer than others do, and that often these differences are closely associated with social characteristics such as race, ethnicity, gender, location, and socioeconomic status."[50] These gaps between groups have been referred to as *health disparities* (also call health inequalities in some countries). More formally, **health disparities** has been defined as the difference in health among different populations. Health disparities are a problem in the United States in that many minority groups' health status, on many different measures, is not as good as the white population. Efforts have been put forth to eliminate the disparities, as evidenced by one of the *Healthy People 2020* overarching goals to "achieve health equity, eliminate disparities, and improve the health for all groups." Many experts think these differences have been caused by two *health inequities*—lack of access to health care, and/or when health care is received the quality has not been as good for those in minority groups. Whatever the reason, health disparities continue to be a problem and much more needs to be done.

Disasters

Disasters can be classified into two primary categories—natural (or conventional) and humanmade (or technological disasters).[1] Whereas *natural disasters* are the result of the combination of the forces of nature (e.g., hurricane, flood, blizzard, tornado, earthquake, landslide) and human activities,[51] *humanmade disasters* result from either unintentional (e.g., spill of a toxic substance into the environment) or intentional (e.g., bioterrorism) human activities, often associated with the use or misuse of technology. Both types of disasters have the potential to cause injury, death, disease, and damage to property on a large scale.[1] In recent years, the United States has felt the large-scale impact of both types of disasters via the Gulf oil spill, Hurricanes Katrina and Rita, and the severe flooding in the middle of the country. All of these events showed us that the preparation for such disasters was not adequate and that each type of disaster required different resources and a different response.

Even though the causes of the two categories of disasters are different, preparedness for them has many common elements. It has been noted that preparedness for natural disasters is the foundation for preparedness for humanmade disasters.[52] That is, in preparing for natural disasters, the basic components of an adequate disaster response system have been defined, and the steps necessary to build disaster preparedness capacity have been established.[52] What needs to be added are specific steps to deal with the peculiarity of the humanmade disasters. An example of this would be the need for decontamination following exposure to a biological agent.

Content removed due to copyright restrictions

Even given the devastating consequences of natural disasters, such as Hurricanes Katrina and Rita, flooding, or the forest fires that consume many thousands of acres of woodlands each year, it has been the intentional humanmade disasters—specifically terrorism—that have occupied much of our attention in recent years (see Figure 9).

Mention was made earlier of the use of a communicable disease as part of terrorism. However, in fact a number of agents could be used as part of terrorism. Since the anthrax mailings, community and public health professionals have focused on the possibility that future terrorism could include chemical, nuclear/radiological, and/or biological (CNB) agents, resulting in mass numbers of casualties. Such concern led to an evaluation of community and public health emergency preparedness and response. "Determining the level of state and local health departments' emergency preparedness and response capacities is crucial because public health officials are among those, along with firefighters, emergency medical personnel, and local law enforcement personnel, who serve on 'rapid response' teams when large-scale emergency situations arise."[13] Results of that evaluation showed that the public health infrastructure was not where it should be to handle large-scale emergencies, as well as a number of more common public health concerns.

public health preparedness the ability of the *public health system, community, and individuals* to prevent, protect against, quickly respond to, and recover from health emergencies, particularly those in which scale, timing, or unpredictability threatens to overwhelm routine capabilities

> The . . . public health infrastructure has suffered from political neglect and from the pressure of political agendas and public opinion that frequently override empirical evidence. Under the glare of a national crisis, policy makers and the public became aware of vulnerable and outdated health information systems and technologies, an insufficient and inadequately trained public health workforce, antiquated laboratory capacity, a lack of real-time surveillance and epidemiological systems, ineffective and fragmented communications networks, incomplete domestic preparedness and emergency response capabilities, and communities without access to essential public health services.[13]

medical preparedness the ability of the *health care system* to prevent, protect against, quickly respond to, and recover from health emergencies, particularly those whose scale, timing, or unpredictability threatens to overwhelm routine capabilities

Based on the results of several different evaluations that exposed many weaknesses in emergency preparedness in general and in the public health infrastructure more specifically, investment in public health preparedness has increased since September 11, 2001. Those federal departments that have been responsible for most of the effort have been the Departments of Homeland Security (DHS) and Health and Human Services (DHHS). The DHS has the responsibility of protecting America, whereas the DHHS, has taken the leadership for public health and medical preparedness. **Public health preparedness** has been defined as "the ability of the *public health system, community, and individuals* to prevent, protect against, quickly respond to, and recover from health emergencies, particularly those in which scale, timing, or unpredictability threatens to overwhelm routine capabilities,"[53] and **medical preparedness** has been defined as "the ability of the *health care system* to prevent, protect against, quickly respond to, and recover from health emergencies, particularly those whose scale, timing, or unpredictability threatens to overwhelm routine capabilities."[53] Information about emergency preparedness and response can be found on the Web sites of all DHHS agencies; however, those that have been most visible have been the Centers for Disease Control and Prevention (CDC), the Health Resources and Services Administration (HRSA), and the Agency for Healthcare Research and Quality (AHRQ).

Since 9/11, the federal government, through a variety of funding sources and programs, has worked to strengthen homeland security, emergency preparedness, and response at all levels. The funding has been used to create or enhance the various components needed in disaster situations (i.e., communication, coordination, and training for personnel). The funding also had to be used to bring much of the public health system up-to-date (i.e., laboratories, personnel, and surveillance) after many years of neglect.

Though the United States is better prepared than prior to 9/11, much still needs to be done. In December 2009, the Trust for America's Health (TFAH), a nonprofit, nonpartisan organization, and the Robert Wood Johnson Foundation released their seventh report on the state of public health preparedness in the United States.[54] The report, titled *Ready or Not 2009?: Protecting the Public's Health from Disease, Disasters, and Bioterrrorism*, contained preparedness scores for all 50 states and the District of Columbia based on 10 key indicators to assess health emergency preparedness capabilities. Much of the seventh report focuses on the H1N1 flu outbreak the previous flu season. The indicators were developed in consultation with leading public health experts based on data from publicly available sources or information provided by public officials. "Twenty states scored six or less out of 10 key indicators of public health emergency preparedness. Nearly two-thirds of states scored seven or less. Eight states tied for the highest score of nine out of 10: Arkansas, Delaware, New York, North Carolina, North Dakota, Oklahoma, Texas, and Vermont. Montana had the lowest score at three out of 10."[54] Some key findings from the report include the following:

- 27 states cut funding for public health from FY 2007–08 to 2008–09.
- 13 states have purchased less than 50 percent of their share of federally subsidized antiviral drugs to stockpile for use during an influenza pandemic.
- 14 states do not have the capacity in place to assure the timely pick-up and delivery of laboratory samples on a 24/7 basis to the Laboratory Response Network (LRN).
- 11 states and D.C. report not having enough laboratory staffing capacity to work five 12-hour days for six to eight weeks in response to an infectious disease outbreak, such as H1N1.[54]

Michelle Larkin, JD, Public Health Team Director and Senior Program Officer at the Robert Wood Johnson Foundation, commented on the report by saying, "State and local health departments around the country are being asked to do more with less during the H1N1 outbreak as budgets continue to be stretched beyond their limits. Public health provides essential prevention and preparedness services that help us lead healthier lives—without sustained and stable funding, Americans will continue to be needlessly at risk from the next public health threat."[55]

Outlook for Community Health in the Twenty-First Century

So far in this chapter we have discussed community health, past and present. Now we describe what community health leaders in the United States and elsewhere in the world hope to achieve in the coming years.

World Planning for the Twenty-First Century

World health leaders recognized the need to plan for the twenty-first century at the thirtieth World Health Assembly of the World Health Organization, held in 1977. At that assembly, delegations from governments around the world set as a target "that the level of health to be attained by the turn of the century should be that which will permit all people to lead a socially and economically productive life."[56] This target goal became known as "Health for All by the Year 2000." The following year in Alma-Ata, U.S.S.R., the joint WHO/UNICEF (United Nations Children's Fund) International Conference adopted a Declaration on Primary Health Care as the key to attaining the goal of Health for All by the Year 2000. At the thirty-fourth World Health Assembly in 1981, delegates from the member nations unanimously adopted a Global Strategy for Health for All by the Year 2000. That same year, the United Nations General Assembly endorsed the Global Strategy and urged other international organizations concerned with community health to collaborate with the WHO. The underlying concept of Health for All by the Year 2000 was that health resources should be distributed in such a way that essential health care services are accessible to everyone.

As we now know, the lofty goal of health for all around the world by the year 2000 was not reached. That does not mean that the goal was abandoned. With the passing into a new century, the program was renamed Health for All (HFA). HFA continues to seek "to create the conditions where people have, as a fundamental human right, the opportunity to reach and maintain the highest level of health. The vision of a renewed HFA policy builds on the WHO Constitution, the experience of the past and the needs for the future."[57]

As one might expect with all of the unrest worldwide, the progress to HFA is slow. Yet, some progress has been made. Life expectancy has increased by between 6 and 7 years globally in the last 30 years, due primarily to (1) social and economic development, (2) the wider provision of safe water and sanitation facilities, and (3) the expansion of national health services.[58] However, all do not share in this increased life expectancy. "There are widening health inequities between and within countries, between rich and poor, between men and women, and between different ethnic groups. More than a billion of the world's poorest people are not benefiting from the major advances in health care and several countries, particularly in sub-Saharan Africa, have seen a decline in life expectancy due in part to the HIV/AIDS epidemic."[58]

The work and the related tasks that face the WHO are enormous. The widening health gap is fueled by the impact of communicable diseases, global increases in noncommunicable diseases (especially from tobacco use, unhealthy diets, physical inactivity, and alcohol abuse), and unintentional injuries (primarily from road traffic crashes). What makes the work even more difficult is that "WHO operates in an increasingly complex and rapidly changing landscape. The boundaries of public health action have become blurred, extending into other sectors that influence health opportunities and outcomes. WHO responds to these challenges using a six-point agenda. The six points address two health objectives, two strategic needs, and two operational approaches."[59] These six points and a brief rationale for each are presented in Box 4.

As might be inferred from the stated priority areas in Box 4, much of the attention for improved world health in the twenty-first century is focused on the less developed and poorer countries of the world. The plan for tackling these global health challenges and other non-health-related global challenges of the twenty-first century is guided by the *United Nations Millennium Declaration*,[60] which was adopted at the United Nations' Millennium Summit in September 2000. More information about the declaration is presented in the section that discusses the WHO.

Content removed due to

copyright restrictions

The United States' Planning for the Twenty-First Century

In addition to its participation in WHO's plans for the twenty-first century, the United States has created its own plans. The United States has decided to develop its planning process around 10-year blocks of time. The current plan is called *Healthy People 2020*.[61] As noted earlier in this chapter, *Healthy People 2020* and its three predecessor editions do in fact outline the health agenda of the nation. Some have referred to the *Healthy People* documents as the health blueprint of the nation. Each of these documents obviously is created on the best available data at the time, but all have been structured in a similar way. All four editions include several overarching goals and many supporting objectives for the nation's health. The goals provide a general focus and direction, while the objectives are used to measure progress within a specified period of time. Formal reviews (i.e., measured progress) of these objectives are conducted both at midcourse (i.e., halfway through the 10-year period) and again at the end of 10 years. The midcourse review provides an opportunity to update the document based on the events of the first half of the decade for which the objectives are written. For example, in *Healthy People 2010*, a number of objectives were changed, updated, or deleted because of the events of 9/11 and Hurricanes Katrina and Rita. Both the results of the midcourse and end reviews along with other available data are used to help create the next set of goals and objectives.

Healthy People 2020, which was released in December 2010, includes a vision statement, a mission statement, four overarching goals (see Table 2), and many objectives spread over 42 different topic areas (see Table 3). On the Healthy People.gov Web site each topic has its own Web page. At a minimum each page contains a concise goal statement, a brief overview of the topic that provides the background and context for the topic, a statement about the importance of the topic backed up by appropriate evidence, and references. There are two types of objectives—measurable and developmental. The measurable objectives provide direction for action and include national baseline data from which the 2020 target was set. The developmental objectives provide a vision for a desired outcome or health status, but national baseline data were not available when they were written. The purpose of developmental objectives is to identify areas of emerging importance and to drive the development of data systems to measure them.

The developers of *Healthy People 2020* think that the best way to implement the national objectives is with the framework referred to as MAP-IT (see Figure 10). MAP-IT stands for Mobilize, Assess, Plan, Implement, and Track. The Mobilize step of MAP-IT deals with bringing interested parties together within communities to deal with health issues. The second step, Assess, is used to find out who is affected by the health problem and examine what resources are available to deal with the problem. In the Plan step, goals and objectives are created and an intervention is planned that has the best chances of dealing with the health problem. The Implement step deals with putting the intervention into action. And the final step, Track, deals with evaluating the impact of the intervention on the health problem.[61]

Table 2
***Healthy People 2020* Vision, Mission, and Goals**

Vision

A society in which all people live long, healthy lives.

Mission

Healthy People 2020 strives to:

- Identify nationwide health improvement priorities
- Increase public awareness and understanding of the determinants of health, disease, and disability and the opportunities for progress
- Provide measurable objectives and goals that are applicable at the national, state, and local levels
- Engage multiple sectors to take actions to strengthen policies and improve practices that are driven by the best available evidence and knowledge
- Identify critical research, evaluation, and data collection needs

Overarching Goals

- Attain high-quality, longer lives free of preventable disease, disability, injury, and premature death.
- Achieve health equity, eliminate disparities, and improve the health of all groups.
- Create social and physical environments that promote good health for all.
- Promote quality of life, healthy development, and healthy behaviors across all life stages.

Source: U.S. Department of Health and Human Services (2010). *About Healthy People*. Available at http://www.healthypeople.gov/2020/about/default.aspx. Accessed December 13, 2010.

Table 3
***Healthy People 2020* Topic Areas**

1. Access to Health Services	21. Heart Disease and Stroke
2. Adolescent Health	22. HIV
3. Arthritis, Osteoporosis, and Chronic Back Conditions	23. Immunization and Infectious Diseases
4. Blood Disorders and Blood Safety	24. Injury and Violence Prevention
5. Cancer	25. Lesbian, Gay, Bisexual, and Transgender Health
6. Chronic Kidney Disease	26. Maternal, Infant, and Child Health
7. Dementias, Including Alzheimer's Disease	27. Medical Product Safety
8. Diabetes	28. Mental Health and Mental Disorders
9. Disability and Health	29. Nutrition and Weight Status
10. Early and Middle Childhood	30. Occupational Safety and Health
11. Educational and Community-Based Programs	31. Older Adults
12. Environmental Health	32. Oral Health
13. Family Planning	33. Physical Activity
14. Food Safety	34. Preparedness
15. Genomics	35. Public Health Infrastructure
16. Global Health	36. Respiratory Diseases
17. Healthcare-Associated Infections	37. Sexually Transmitted Diseases
18. Health Communication and Health Information Technology	38. Sleep Health
19. Health-Related Quality of Life and Well-Being	39. Social Determinants of Health
20. Hearing and Other Sensory or Communication Disorders	40. Substance Abuse
	41. Tobacco Use
	42. Vision

Source: U.S. Department of Health and Human Services (2010). *Topics & Objectives Index—Healthy People*. Available at http://www.healthypeople.gov/2020/topicsobjectives2020/default.aspx. Accessed December 13, 2010.

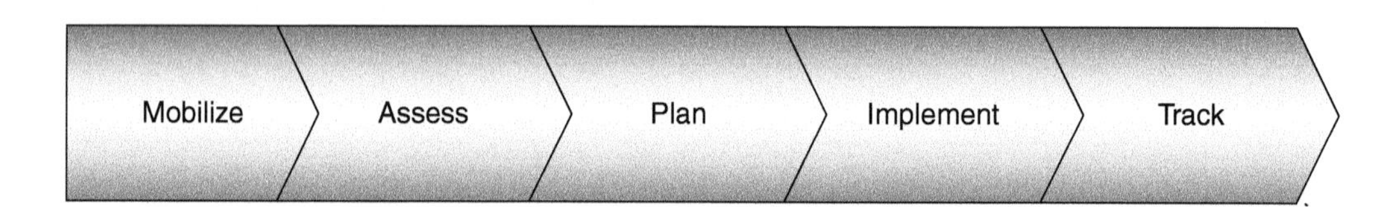

FIGURE 10

The Action Model to Achieve Healthy People Goals

Source: U.S. Department of Health and Human Services (2010). *Implementing Healthy People 2020*. Available at http://www.healthypeople.gov/2020/implementing/default.aspx. Accessed December 16, 2010.

As can be seen in the material presented in the last few pages, both the World Health Organization and the U.S. Department of Health and Human Services have much work ahead to improve the health of the people of the world and the United States in the twenty-first century. Because the planning to improve health is always changing, we urge all students of community and public health to stay up-to-date by regularly visiting both the World Health Organization and *Healthy People 2020* Web sites.

Chapter Summary

- A number of key terms are associated with the study of community health, including *health, community, community health, population health, public health, public health system,* and *global health.*
- The four factors that affect the health of a community are physical (e.g., community size), social and cultural (e.g., religion), community organization, and individual behaviors (e.g., exercise and diet).
- It is important to be familiar with and understand the history of community health to be able to deal with the present and future community health issues.
- The earliest community health practices went unrecorded; however, archeological findings of ancient societies (before 500 B.C.) show evidence of concern for community health. There is evidence during the time of the classical cultures (500 B.C.–A.D. 500) that people were interested in physical strength, medicine, and sanitation.
- The belief of many living during the Middle Ages (A.D. 500–1500) was that health and disease were associated with spirituality. Many epidemics were seen during this period.
- During the Renaissance period (A.D. 1500–1700), there was a growing belief that disease was caused by the environment, not spiritual factors.
- The eighteenth century was characterized by industrial growth. Science was being used more in medicine and it was during this century that the first vaccine was discovered.
- The nineteenth century ushered in the modern era of public health. The germ theory was introduced during this time, and the last fourth of the century is known as the bacteriological period of public health.
- The twentieth century can be divided into several periods. The health resources development period (1900–1960) was a time when many public and private resources were used to improve health. The period of social engineering (1960–1973) saw the U.S. government's involvement in health insurance through Medicare and Medicaid. The health promotion period began in 1974 and continues today.
- Great concern still exists for health care, the environment, diseases caused by an impoverished lifestyle, the spread of communicable diseases (such as AIDS, Legionnaires' disease, toxic shock syndrome, and Lyme disease), the harm caused by alcohol and other drug abuse, and terrorism.
- Both the WHO and the U.S. government continue to plan for the health of humanity. The planning of the United States is reflected in the *Healthy People* documents, the health agenda for the nation.

Scenario: Analysis and Response

The Internet has many sources of information that could help Amy and Eric with the decisions that they will have to make about the continued use of the day care center for their children. Use a search engine (e.g., Google, Bing) and enter (a) hepatitis, and (b) hepatitis and day care centers. Print out the information that you find and use it in answering the following questions.

1. Based on the information you found on the Web, if you were Amy or Eric would you take your children to the day care center the next day? Why or why not?
2. Do you feel the hepatitis problem in day care centers is a personal health concern or a community health concern? Why?
3. Which of the factors noted in this chapter that affect the health of a community play a part in the hepatitis problem faced by Amy and Eric?
4. Why does the hepatitis problem remind us of the health problems faced by people in this country prior to 1900?
5. Under which of the focus areas in the *Healthy People 2020* would hepatitis fall? Why?

Review Questions

1. How did the WHO define health in 1946? How has that definition been modified?
2. What is public health?
3. What are the differences among community health, population health, and global health?
4. What are the five major domains that determine a person's health?
5. What is the difference between personal health activities and community health activities?
6. Define the term *community*.
7. What are four major factors that affect the health of a community? Provide an example of each.
8. Identify some of the major events of community health in each of the following periods of time:

   Early civilizations (prior to A.D. 500)

   Middle Ages (A.D. 500–1500)

   Renaissance and Exploration (A.D. 1500–1700)

   The eighteenth century

   The nineteenth century
9. Provide a brief explanation of the origins from which the following twentieth-century periods get their names:

   Health resources development period

   Period of social engineering

   Period of health promotion
10. What are the major community health problems facing the United States in the twenty-first century?
11. What is included in the World Health Organization's Agenda?
12. What significance do the *Healthy People* documents have in community health development in recent years?
13. What significance do you think *Healthy People 2020* will have in the years ahead?

Activities

1. Write your own definition for *health*.
2. In a two-page paper, explain how the five major determinants of health could interact to cause a disease such as cancer.
3. In a one-page paper, explain why heart disease can be both a personal health problem and a community health problem.
4. Select a community health problem that exists in your hometown; then, using the factors that affect the health of a community noted in this chapter, analyze and discuss in a two-page paper at least three factors that contribute to the problem in your hometown.
5. Select one of the following individuals (all have been identified in this chapter), go to the library and do some additional reading or find two reliable Web sites, and then write a two-page paper on the person's contribution to community health.

   Edward Jenner

   John Snow

   Lemuel Shattuck

   Louis Pasteur

   Robert Koch

   Walter Reed
6. Review a copy of *Healthy People 2020* on the Web. Then, set up a time to talk with an administrator in your hometown health department. Find out which of the objectives the health department has been working on as priorities. Summarize in a paper what the objectives are, what the health department is doing about them, and what it hopes to accomplish by the year 2020.

Community Health on the Web

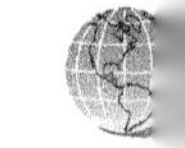

The Internet contains a wealth of information about community and public health. Increase your knowledge of some of the topics presented in this chapter by accessing the Jones & Bartlett Learning Web site at **http://health.jbpub.com/book/communityhealth/7e** and follow the links to complete the following Web activities.

- *Healthy People 2020*
- Department of Homeland Security
- Global Health

References

1. Schneider, M.-J. (2011). *Introduction to Public Health*, 3rd ed. Sudbury, MA: Jones and Bartlett.
2. Bunker, J. P., H. S. Frazier, and F. Mosteller (1994). "Improving Health: Measuring Effects of Medical Care." *Milbank Quarterly*, 72: 225–258.
3. Centers for Disease Control and Prevention (1999). "Ten Great Public Health Achievements—United States, 1900–1999." *Morbidity and Mortality Weekly Report*, 48(12): 241–243.
4. Koplan, J. (2000). *21st Century Health Challenges: Can We All Become Healthy, Wealthy, and Wise?* Available at http://www.pitt.edu/~super1/lecture/lec1361/origin.htm.
5. National Safety Council (1997). *Accident Facts, 1997 Edition*. Itasca, IL: Author.
6. World Health Organization (2010). *Glossary of Globalization, Trade, and Health Terms*. Geneva, Switzerland: Author. Available at http://www.who.int/trade/glossary/en/.
7. Hancock, T., and M. Minkler (2005). "Community Health Assessment or Healthy Community Assessment." In M. Minkler, ed., *Community Organizing and Community Building for Health*, 2nd ed. New Brunswick, NJ: Rutgers University Press, 138–157.

8. McGinnis, J. M. (2001). "United States." In C. E. Koop, ed., *Critical Issues in Global Health*. San Francisco: Jossey-Bass, 80-90.

9. McGinnis, J. M., P. Williams-Russo, and J. R. Knickman (2002). "The Case for More Active Policy Attention to Health Promotion." *Health Affairs*, 21(2): 78-93.

10. Turnock, B. J. (2009). *Public Health: What It Is and How It Works*, 4th ed. Sudbury, MA: Jones and Bartlett.

11. Minkler, M., N. Wallerstein, and N. Wilson (2008). "Improving Health Through Community Organizing and Community Building." In K. Glanz, B. K. Rimer, and K. Viswanath, eds., *Health Behavior and Health Education Practice: Theory, Research, and Practice*, 4th ed. San Francisco: Jossey-Bass, 287-312.

12. Israel, B. A., B. Checkoway, A. Schulz, and M. Zimmerman (1994). "Health Education and Community Empowerment: Conceptualizing and Measuring Perceptions of Individual, Organizational, and Community Control." *Health Education Quarterly*, 21(2): 149-170.

13. Institute of Medicine (2003). *The Future of the Public's Health in the 21st Century*. Washington, DC: National Academies Press.

14. Institute of Medicine (1988). *The Future of Public Health*. Washington, DC: National Academies Press.

15. Green, L. W., and J. F. McKenzie (2002). "Community and Population Health." In L. Breslow, ed., *Encyclopedia of Public Health*. New York: Macmillan Reference USA.

16. Kasier Family Foundation (2009). *Global Health: Background Brief*. Available at http://www.kaiseredu.org/topics_im.asp?imID=1&id=1033.

17. Institute of Medicine (1997). *America's Vital Interest in Global Health: Protecting Our People, Enhancing Our Economy, and Advancing Our International Interests*. Washington, DC: National Academy Press. Available at http://books.nap.edu/openbook.php?record_id=5717&page=R1.

18. Association for the Advancement of Health Education (1994). *Cultural Awareness and Sensitivity: Guidelines for Health Educators*. Reston, VA: Author.

19. U.S. Department of Health and Human Services, Centers for Disease Control and Prevention (2009). "Cigarette Smoking Among Adults and Trends in Smoking Cessation—United States, 2008." *Morbidity and Mortality Weekly Report*, 58(44): 1227-1232. Available at http://www.cdc.gov/mmwr/preview/mmwrhtml/mm5844a2.htm.

20. American College Health Association (2010). *American College Health Association—National College Health Assessment II (ACHA-NCHA II) Fall 2009: Reference Group Executive Summary*. Available at http://www.acha-ncha.org/reports_ACHA-NCHAII.html.

21. Shi, L., and D. A. Singh (2010). *Essentials of the US Health Care System*, 2nd ed. Sudbury, MA: Jones and Bartlett.

22. U.S. Department of Health and Human Services (2000). *Healthy People 2010*. Available at http://www.healthypeople.gov.

23. Minkler, M., and N. Wallerstein (2005). "Improving Health through Community Organizing and Community Building: A Health Education Perspective." In M. Minkler, ed., *Community Organizing and Community Building for Health*, 2nd ed. New Brunswick, NJ: Rutgers University Press, 26-50.

24. Ross, M. G. (1967). *Community Organization: Theory, Principles, and Practice*. New York: Harper & Row.

25. Pickett, G., and J. J. Hanlon (1990). *Public Health: Administration and Practice*, 9th ed. St. Louis, MO: Times Mirror/Mosby.

26. Legon, R. P. (1986). "Ancient Greece." *World Book Encyclopedia*. Chicago, IL: World Book.

27. Rosen, G. (1958). *A History of Public Health*. New York: MD Publications.

28. Burton, L. E., H. H. Smith, and A. W. Nichols (1980). *Public Health and Community Medicine*, 3rd ed. Baltimore: Williams & Wilkins.

29. Woodruff, A. W. (1977). "Benjamin Rush, His Work on Yellow Fever and His British Connections." *American Journal of Tropical Medicine and Hygiene*, 26(5): 1055-1059.

30. Rosen, G. (1975). *Preventive Medicine in the United States, 1900-1975*. New York: Science History Publications.

31. Smillie, W. G. (1955). *Public Health: Its Promise for the Future*. New York: Macmillan.

32. Duffy, J. (1990). *The Sanitarians: A History of American Public Health*. Chicago: University of Illinois Press.

33. Lalonde, M. (1974). *A New Perspective on the Health of Canadians: A Working Document*. Ottawa, Canada: Minister of Health.

34. Green, L. W. (1999). "Health Education's Contributions to the Twentieth Century: A Glimpse through Health Promotion's Rearview Mirror." In J. E. Fielding, L. B. Lave, and B. Starfield, eds., *Annual Review of Public Health*. Palo Alto, CA: Annual Reviews, 67-88.

35. U.S. Department of Health and Human Services, Public Health Service (1980). *Ten Leading Causes of Death in the United States, 1977*. Washington, DC: U.S. Government Printing Office.

36. U.S. Department of Health, Education, and Welfare (1979). *Healthy People: The Surgeon General's Report on Health Promotion and Disease Prevention* (DHEW pub. no. 79-55071). Washington, DC: U.S. Government Printing Office.

37. McKenzie, J. F., B. L. Neiger, and R. Thackeray (2009). *Planning, Implementing, and Evaluating Health Promotion Programs: A Primer*, 5th ed. San Francisco: Benjamin Cummings.

38. U.S. Department of Health and Human Services (1980). *Promoting Health/Preventing Disease: Objectives for the Nation*. Washington, DC: U.S. Government Printing Office.

39. U.S. Department of Health and Human Services, Centers for Medicare and Medicaid Services (2010). *National Health Expenditure Data*. Available at http://www.cms.gov/NationalHealthExpendData/01_Overview.asp#TopOfPage.

40. U.S. Census Bureau (2010). *World Population 1950-2050*. Available at http://www.census.gov/ipc/www/idb/worldpopgraph.php.

41. Miniño, A. M., J. Q. Xu, and K. D. Kochanek (2010). "Deaths: Preliminary Data for 2008." *National Vital Statistics Reports*, 59(2): Hyattsville, MD: National Center for Health Statistics..

42. U.S. Department of Health and Human Services (1990). *Prevention '89/'90*. Washington, DC: U.S. Government Printing Office.

43. Centers for Disease Control (1981). "Pneumocystis Pneumonia—Los Angeles." *Morbidity and Mortality Weekly Report*, 30: 250-252.

44. Centers for Disease Control (1989). "First 100,000 Cases of Acquired Immunodeficiency Syndrome—United States." *Morbidity and Mortality Weekly Report*, 38: 561-563.

45. Centers for Disease Control (1992). "The Second 100,000 Cases of Acquired Immunodeficiency Syndrome—United States, June 1981-December 1991." *Morbidity and Mortality Weekly Report*, 42(2): 28-29.

46. Centers for Disease Control and Prevention (2006). "Twenty-five Years of HIV/AIDS—United States, 1981-2006." *Morbidity and Mortality Weekly Report*, 55(21): 585-589.

47. Centers for Disease Control and Prevention (2010). *Diagnoses of HIV Infection and AIDS in the United States and Dependent Areas: 2008 HIV Surveillance Report*. Available at http://www.cdc.gov/hiv/surveillance/resources/reports/2008report/.

48. Gerberding, J. L., J. M. Hughes, and J. P. Koplan (2003). "Bioterrorism Preparedness and Response: Clinicians and Public Health Agencies as Essential Partners." In P. R. Lee and C. L. Estes, eds., *The Nation's Health*. Sudbury, MA: Jones and Bartlett, 305-309.

49. Pinger, R. R., W. A. Payne, D. B. Hahn, and E. J. Hahn (1998). *Drugs: Issues for Today*, 3rd ed. Boston: WCB McGraw-Hill.

50. King, N. (2009). "Health Inequalities and Health Inequities." In E. E. Morrison, ed., *Health Care Ethics: Critical Issues for the 21st Century*. Sudbury, MA: Jones and Bartlett, 339-354

51. Federal Emergency Management Agency (2007). "Are You Ready? Natural Disaster." Available at http://www.fema.gov/areyouready/natural_hazards.shtm.

52. Agency for Healthcare Research and Quality (2004). *Bioterrorism and Health System Preparedness* (Issue Brief no. 2). Available at http://www.ahrq.gov/news/ulp/btbriefs/btbrief2.htm.

53. Centers for Disease Control and Prevention (2010). *Emergency Preparedness and Response: What CDC Is Doing*. Available at http://www.bt.cdc.gov/cdc/.

54. Trust for America's Health and the Robert Wood Johnson Foundation (2009). *Ready or Not 2009?: Protecting the Public's Health from Disease, Disasters, and Bioterrorism*. Available at http://healthyamericans.org/reports/bioterror09/.

55. Trust for America's Health (2009). *New Report: H1N1 Reveals Gaps in Nation's Emergency Health Preparedness Efforts; Twenty States Score Six or Less Out of Ten Key Indicators*. Press release. Available at http://healthyamericans.org/newsroom/releases/?releaseid=201.

56. World Health Organization (1990). *Facts about WHO*. Geneva, Switzerland: Author.

57. World Health Organization (2003). *World Health Report 2003: Shaping the Future*. Geneva, Switzerland: Author.

58. World Healt=h Organization (2006). *Engaging in Health: Eleventh General Programme of Work 2006-2015*. Available at http://www.whyqlibdoc.who.int.hq/2006/GPW_ES_2006-2015_eng.pdf.

59. World Health Organization (2010). *The WHO Agenda*. Available at http://www.who.int/about/agenda/en/index.html.

60. United Nations (2000). *United Nations Millennium Declaration*. New York: Author.

61. U.S. Department of Health and Human Services (2010). *Implementing Healthy People 2020*. Available at http://www.healthypeople.gov/2020/implementing/default.aspx.

PHOTO CREDITS

Opener Hannus Design Associates

2 © Rubberball Productions/Getty Images; **3** © Weldon Schloneger/ShutterStock, Inc.; **4** © Styve Reineck/ShutterStock, Inc.; **5** Courtesy of Dr. John Noble, Jr./CDC; **7** Courtesy of Library of Congress, Prints & Photographs Division, [reproduction number LC-USZ62-7386]; **8** © coka/ShutterStock, Inc.;

Unless otherwise indicated, all photographs and illustrations are under copyright of Jones & Bartlett Learning, or have been provided by the authors.

Organizations That Help Shape Community Health

Chapter Outline

Chapter Objectives

After studying this chapter, you will be able to:

1. Explain the need for organizing to improve community health.
2. Explain what a governmental health organization is and give an example of one at each of the following levels—international, national, state, and local.
3. Explain the role the World Health Organization (WHO) plays in community health.
4. Briefly describe the structure and function of the United States Department of Health and Human Services (HHS).
5. State the three core functions of public health.
6. List the 10 essential public health services.
7. Explain the relationship between a state and local health department.
8. Explain what is meant by the term *coordinated school health program.*
9. Define the term *quasi-governmental* and explain why some health organizations are classified under this term.
10. List the four primary activities of most voluntary health organizations.
11. Explain the purpose of a professional health organization/association.
12. Explain how philanthropic foundations contribute to community health.
13. Discuss the role that service, social, and religious organizations play in community health.
14. Identify the major reason why corporations are involved in community health and describe some corporate activities that contribute to community health.

SCENARIO

Mary is a hardworking senior at the local university. She is majoring in physical education and looking forward to teaching elementary physical education after graduation. Mary has always been involved in team sports and has been a lifeguard at the local swimming pool for the past 4 years. Mary has a fair complexion with honey-blonde hair and blue eyes. She has always tanned easily, so, has not bothered very much with sunscreens. For the past few weeks, Mary has noticed a red, scaly, sharply outlined patch of skin on her forehead. She has put creams and ointments on it, but it will not go away and may be getting larger. Her roommate, Clare, suggests that she should make an appointment with the campus health services office. Mary lets it go another week and then decides to see the doctor.

After looking at the patch of skin, the doctor refers Mary to a specialist, Dr. Rice, who is a dermatologist. The dermatologist suggests a biopsy be taken of the lesion to test for skin cancer. The specialist tells Mary that if it is cancer, it is probably still in its early stages and so the prognosis is good.

A potential diagnosis of cancer often raises a lot of questions and concerns. Are there any resources in the community to which Mary can turn for help?

INTRODUCTION

The history of community health dates to antiquity. For much of that history, community health issues were addressed only on an emergency basis. For example, if a community faced a drought or an epidemic, a town meeting would be called to deal with the problem. It has been only in the last 100 years or so that communities have taken explicit actions to deal aggressively with health issues on a continual basis.

Today's communities differ from those of the past in several important ways. Although individuals are better educated, more mobile, and more independent than in the past, communities are less autonomous and are more dependent on state and federal funding for support. Contemporary communities are too large and complex to respond effectively to sudden health emergencies or to make long-term improvements in public health without community organization and careful planning. Better community organizing and careful long-term planning are essential to ensure that a community makes the best use of its resources for health, both in times of emergency and over the long run.

The ability of today's communities to respond effectively to their own problems is hindered by the following characteristics: (1) highly developed and centralized resources in our national institutions and organizations, (2) continuing concentration of wealth and population in the largest metropolitan areas, (3) rapid movement of information, resources, and people made possible by advanced communication and transportation technologies that eliminate the need for local offices where resources were once housed, (4) the globalization of health, (5) limited horizontal relationships between/among organizations, and (6) a system of **top-down funding** (money that comes from either the federal or state government to the local level) for many community programs.[1]

top-down funding a method of funding in which funds are transmitted from federal or state government to the local level

In this chapter, we discuss organizations that help to shape a community's ability to respond effectively to health-related issues by protecting and promoting the health of the community and its members. These community organizations can be classified as governmental, quasi-governmental, and nongovernmental—according to their sources of funding, responsibilities, and organizational structure.

Governmental Health Agencies

Governmental health agencies are part of the governmental structure (federal, state, or local). They are funded primarily by tax dollars and managed by government officials. Each governmental health agency is designated as having authority over some geographic area. Such agencies exist at the four governmental levels—international, national, state, and local.

governmental health agencies health agencies that are part of the governmental structure (federal, state, or local) and that are funded primarily by tax dollars

International Health Agencies

The most widely recognized international governmental health organization today is the **World Health Organization (WHO)** (see Figure 1). Its headquarters is located in Geneva, Switzerland, and there are six regional offices around the world. The names, acronyms, and cities and countries of location for WHO regional offices are as follows: Africa (AFRO), Brazzaville, Congo; Americas (PAHO), Washington, DC, United States; Eastern Mediterranean (EMRO), Cairo, Egypt; Europe (EURO), Copenhagen, Denmark; Southeast Asia (SEARO), New Delhi, India; and Western Pacific (WPRO), Manila, Philippines.[2]

World Health Organization (WHO) the most widely recognized international governmental health organization

Although the WHO is now the largest international health organization, it is not the oldest. Among the organizations (listed with their founding dates) that predate WHO are the following:

- International D'Hygiene Publique (1907), which was absorbed by the WHO;
- the Health Organization of the League of Nations (1919), which was dissolved when the WHO was created;
- the United Nations Relief and Rehabilitation Administration (1943) was dissolved in 1946, and its work is carried out today by the Office of the United Nations High Commissioner for Refugees (UNHCR) (1950);
- the United Nations Children's Fund (UNICEF) (1946) which was formerly known as the United Nations International Children's Emergency Fund;
- and the Pan American Health Organization (PAHO) (1902), which is still an independent organization but is integrated with WHO in a regional office.

Because the WHO is the largest and most visible international health agency, it is discussed at greater length in the following sections.

History of the World Health Organization

Planning for the WHO began when a charter of the United Nations was adopted at an international meeting in 1945. Contained in the charter was an article calling for the establishment of a health agency with wide powers. In 1946, at the International Health Conference, representatives from all of the countries in the United Nations succeeded in creating and ratifying the constitution of the WHO. However, it was not until April 7, 1948, that the constitution went into force and the organization officially began its work. In recognition of this beginning, April 7 is commemorated each year as World Health Day.[2] The sixtieth anniversary of the WHO was celebrated in 2008.

Organization of the World Health Organization

Membership in the WHO is open to any nation that has ratified the WHO constitution and receives a majority vote of the World Health Assembly. At the beginning of 2010, 193 countries were members.

World Health Assembly
a body of delegates of the member nations of the WHO

The **World Health Assembly** comprises the delegates of the member nations. This assembly, which meets in general sessions annually and in special sessions when necessary, has the primary tasks of approving the WHO program and the budget for the following biennium and deciding major policy questions.[2]

The WHO is administered by a staff that includes a director-general, deputy director-general, and nine assistant directors-general. Great care is taken to ensure political balance in staffing WHO positions, particularly at the higher levels of administration.

Purpose and Work of the World Health Organization

The primary objective of the WHO, as stated in the constitution, is the attainment by all peoples of the highest possible level of health.[2] To achieve this objective, the WHO has 22 core functions:

- Act as the directing and coordinating authority on international health work
- Establish and maintain effective collaboration with the United Nations, specialized agencies, governmental health administrations, professional groups, and such other organizations as may be deemed appropriate
- Assist governments, upon request, in strengthening health services
- Furnish appropriate technical assistance and, in emergencies, necessary aid upon the request or acceptance of governments
- Provide or assist in providing, upon the request of the United Nations, health services and facilities to special groups, such as the peoples of trust territories
- Establish and maintain such administrative and technical services as may be required, including epidemiologic and statistical services
- Stimulate and advance work to eradicate epidemic, endemic, and other diseases
- Promote, in cooperation with other specialized agencies where necessary, the prevention of accidental injuries
- Promote, in cooperation with other specialized agencies where necessary, the improvement of nutrition, housing, sanitation, recreation, economic or working conditions, and other aspects of environmental hygiene
- Promote cooperation among scientific and professional groups that contribute to the advancement of health
- Propose conventions, agreements, and regulations and make recommendations with respect to international health matters and perform such duties as may be assigned thereby to the WHO that are consistent with its objective
- Promote maternal and child health and welfare and foster the ability to live harmoniously in a changing total environment
- Foster activities in the field of mental health, especially those affecting the harmony of human relations
- Promote and conduct research in the field of health
- Promote improved standards of teaching and training in the health, medical, and related professions
- Study and report on, in cooperation with other specialized agencies, where necessary, administrative and social techniques affecting public health and medical care from preventive and curative points of view, including hospital services and social security
- Provide information, counsel, and assistance in the field of health

- Assist in developing an informed public opinion among all peoples on matters of health
- Establish and revise as necessary international nomenclatures of diseases, of causes of death, and of public health practices
- Standardize diagnostic procedures as necessary
- Develop, establish, and promote international standards with respect to food, biological, pharmaceutical, and similar products
- Generally, take all necessary action to attain the objective of the organization[2]

The work of the WHO is financed by its member nations, each of which is assessed according to its ability to pay; the wealthiest countries contribute the greatest portion of the total budget.

Although the WHO has sponsored and continues to sponsor many worthwhile programs, an especially noteworthy one was the work of the WHO in helping to eradicate smallpox. In 1967, smallpox was active in 31 countries. During that year, 10 million to 15 million people contracted the disease, and of those, approximately 2 million died and many millions of others were permanently disfigured or blinded. The last known case of smallpox was diagnosed on October 26, 1977, in Somalia.[2] In 1979, the World Health Assembly declared the global eradication of this disease. Using the smallpox mortality figures from 1967, it can be estimated that more than 40 million lives have been saved since the eradication.

More recently, the WHO has made notable achievements in global public health. May 21, 2003, marked the unanimous decision by the World Health Assembly for the WHO to adopt the first global public health treaty to reduce tobacco-related deaths and diseases throughout the world. Additionally, in 2004, the WHO adopted the Global Strategy on Diet, Physical Activity, and Health.

The current work of the WHO is guided by two documents—the *11th General Programme of Work*[2] and the United Nations Millennium Declaration, which was adopted at the Millennium Summit in 2003.[4] Because much of what is included in the *11th General Programme of Work* is summarized in Box 1.4 (The WHO Agenda), the discussion here focuses on the Millennium Declaration. The declaration set out principles and values in seven areas (peace, security, and disarmament; development and poverty eradication; protecting our common environment; human rights, democracy, and good governance; protecting the vulnerable; meeting special needs of Africa; and strengthening the United Nations) that should govern international relations in the twenty-first century.[4] Following the summit, the *Road Map* was prepared, which established goals and targets to be reached by 2015 in each of the seven areas.[5] The resulting eight goals in the area of development and poverty eradication are now referred to as the Millennium Development Goals (MDGs). More specifically, the MDGs are aimed at reducing poverty and hunger, tackling ill health, gender inequality, lack of education, lack of access to clean water, and environmental degradation.

As can be seen from this description, the MDGs are not exclusively aimed at health, but there are interactive processes between health and economic development that create a crucial link. That is, better health is "a prerequisite and major contributor to economic growth and social cohesion. Conversely, improvement in people's access to health technology is a good indicator of the success of other development processes."[3] As such, "three of the eight goals, eight of the 18 targets required to achieve them, and 18 of the 48 indicators of progress are health-related"[3] (see Table 1).

To date, progress has been made to achieve the MDGs by the target date of 2015; however, progress has been, to some extent, relatively slow. The midpoint progress data, evaluated and reported by the United Nations, suggest that some notable progress is being made

Content removed due to

copyright restrictions

even in regions with the greatest challenges.[6] According to The *Millennium Development Goals Report 2007*, "the results achieved in the more successful cases demonstrate that success is possible in most countries, but that the MDGs will be attained only if concerted additional action is taken immediately and sustained until 2015."[6] The following is a summary of achievements documented in the 2007 midpoint progress report:

- Between 1990 and 2004, the proportion of individuals living in extreme poverty reduced from nearly a third to less than one fifth.
- Since 2000, extreme poverty levels for the poor living in sub-Saharan Africa declined by nearly six percentage points; however, it should be noted that the region is not on track to meet the MDG of reducing poverty by half by the target date of 2015.

- Since 1991, primary school enrollment for children in developing countries increased by 8%.
- There has been a slight growth in women's political participation, even in countries where only men were allowed to run for political election. However, progress is very slow.
- Globally, the rate of child mortality has declined.
- Malaria interventions have been expanded.
- The tuberculosis epidemic is on the decline, but not at a rate to reach the 2015 MDG.[6]

Although much progress has been made, there is still much more work to be done. The following lists some of the key challenges, documented by the United Nations, that must be addressed to reach the 2015 MDGs for global health improvement:

- Preventable complications of pregnancy and childbirth take the lives of more than half a million women each year.
- As of 2007, trend projections indicate that the goal of halving the proportion of underweight children will be missed by 30 million children.
- In 2006, AIDS deaths increased to 2.9 million because prevention methods are lacking in keeping pace with the epidemic growth.
- If the 2015 MDG to improve sanitation is to be met, an additional 1.6 billion people will need access to better sanitation (over the 2005–2015 time period).
- Unemployment rates of young people continue to rise.
- Climate change is projected to have serious impact on the progress made toward reaching the MDGs.[6]

Strategies for achieving large-scale and rapid progress toward meeting the MDGs involve strong government leadership and policies and strategies that meet the needs of the poor, combined with sufficient funding and technical support from the international community.[6]

Five major challenges to meeting the goals have been identified: (1) strengthening health systems, (2) ensuring health is recognized as a priority within development and economic policies, (3) developing appropriate strategies to address the diverse needs of the countries, (4) mobilizing more resources for health in the poor countries, and (5) improving the quality of health-related data to track progress toward the goals.[7,8] Much work lies ahead, by all people of the world, to improve the health of those most in need.

National Health Agencies

Each national government has a department or agency that has the primary responsibility for the protection of the health and welfare of its citizens. These national health agencies meet their responsibilities through the development of health policies, the enforcement of health regulations, the provision of health services and programs, the funding of research, and the support of their respective state and local health agencies.

In the United States, the primary national health agency is the Department of Health and Human Services (HHS). HHS "is the United States government's principal agency for protecting the health of all Americans and providing essential human services, especially for those who are least able to help themselves."[9] It is important to note, however, that other federal agencies also contribute to the betterment of our nation's health. For example, the Department of Agriculture inspects meat and dairy products and coordinates the Women, Infants, and Children (WIC) food assistance program; the Environmental Protection Agency (EPA) regulates hazardous wastes; the Department of Labor houses the Occupational

Safety and Health Administration (OSHA), which is concerned with safety and health in the workplace; the Department of Commerce, which includes the Bureau of the Census, collects much of the national data that drive our nation's health programs; and the Department of Homeland Security (DHS) deals with all aspects of terrorism within the United States. Each of these other departments or agencies is discussed in greater detail in later chapters. A detailed description of the Department of Health and Human Services follows.

Department of Health and Human Services

The HHS is headed by the Secretary of Health and Human Services, who is appointed by the president and is a member of his or her cabinet. The Department of Health and Human Services was formed in 1980 (during the administration of President Jimmy Carter), when the Department of Health, Education, and Welfare (HEW) was divided into two new departments, HHS and the Department of Education. HHS is the department most involved with the nation's human concerns. In one way or another it touches the lives of more Americans than any other federal agency. It is literally a department of people serving people, from newborn infants to persons requiring health services to our most elderly citizens. With an annual budget in excess of approximately $707 billion (representing about 25% of the federal budget), HHS is the largest department in the federal government, and it spends approximately $195 billion more per year than the Department of Defense.[9,10]

The fiscal year 2010 overview document of the United States government budget indicated that the approved HHS budget established a reserve fund of more than $630 billion, over a 10-year period, to fund health care system reform. According to the HHS budget document, "the reserve is funded half by new revenue and half by savings proposals that promote efficiency and accountability, align incentives toward quality, and encourage shared responsibility. In addition, the Budget calls for an effort beyond this down payment, to put the Nation on a path to health insurance coverage for all Americans."[10]

To date, some significant legislation has been passed that works toward fundamental health care reform, such as the American Recovery and Reinvestment Act of 2009, which includes $19 billion for health information technology, subsidies for those who are recently unemployed to maintain health insurance, and $1 billion for continued effectiveness research in health.[10] Moreover, in March 2010, a sweeping bill to overhaul the American medical system, put forth by President Barack Obama, was passed by a historic vote of 219 votes to 212. The new health care reform law provided a series of duties and responsibilities for the HHS. Among these were (1) the implementation of new provisions to assist families and small business owners in getting information to make the best choices for insurance coverage, in a "new open, competitive insurance market"; (2) working with states and additional partners to strengthen public programs, such as the children's health insurance plan (CHIP), Medicare, and Medicaid; (3) coordinating efforts with other departments to design and implement "a prevention and health promotion strategy" to promote prevention, wellness, and public health; (4) taking action to strengthen and support the primary care workforce; (5) taking on the new and improved authority to establish a transparent health care system to oversee that every dollar authorized to be spent in the act is done so in a wise and transparent manner; (6) the implementation of new provisions to decrease the costs of medications; (7) taking on authority to establish the Community Living Assistance Services and Supports Act (CLASS Act), which is a voluntary, self-funded long-term-care insurance option; and (8) the implementation of the Indian Health Care Improvement Act (ICHIA), which was reauthorized in the new health care law and provides modernized and improved health care services to Alaska Natives and American Indians.[11]

Since its formation, HHS has undergone several reorganizations. Some of the more recent changes have been the addition of the Center for Faith-Based and Community Initiatives and an Assistant Secretary for Public Health Emergency Preparedness. Currently, the HHS is organized into 11 operating agencies (see Figure 2) whose heads report directly to the Secretary. In addition, the HHS has 10 regional offices (see Table 2). These offices serve as representatives of the Secretary of HHS in direct, official dealings with the state and local governmental organizations. Eight of the 11 operating divisions of HHS (AHRQ, CDC, ATSDR, FDA, HRSA, IHS, NIH, and SAMSHA—see their descriptions below), along with Office of Global Health Affairs (OGHA), the Office of Public Health and Science (OPHS), and the Office

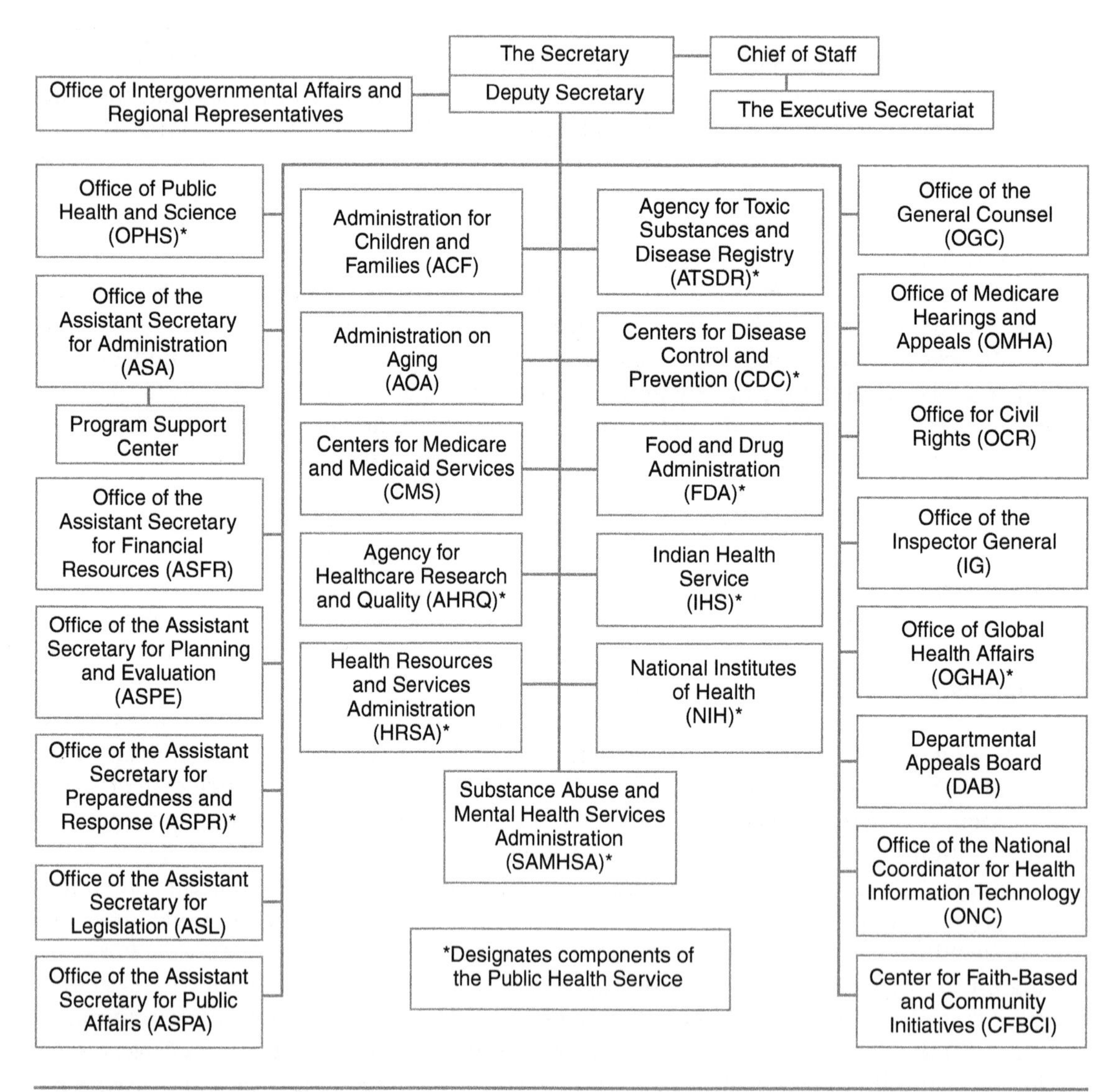

FIGURE 2

Organizational chart for the U.S. Department of Health and Human Services (HHS).

Source: U.S. Department of Health and Human Services (2010). U.S. Department of Health and Human Services Organizational Chart. Available at http://www.hhs.gov/about/orgchart.html. Accessed October 6, 2010.

Table 2
Regional Offices of the U.S. Department of Health and Human Services

Region/Areas Served	Office Address	Telephone Number
Region 1: CT, MA, ME, NH, RI, VT	John F. Kennedy Bldg. Government Center Boston, MA 02203	(617) 565-1500
Region 2: NJ, NY, Puerto Rico, Virgin Islands	Jacob K. Javits Federal Bldg. 26 Federal Plaza New York, NY 10278	(212) 264-4600
Region 3: DE, MD, PA, VA, WV, DC	Public Ledger Building 150 S. Independence Mall West Suite 436 Philadelphia, PA 19106	(215) 861-4633
Region 4: AL, FL, GA, KY, MS, NC, SC, TN	Sam Nunn, Atlanta Federal Center 61 Forsyth Street, SW Atlanta, GA 30303	(404) 562-7888
Region 5: IL, IN, MI, MN, OH, WI	233 N. Michigan Avenue Chicago, IL 60601	(312) 353-5160
Region 6: AR, LA, NM, OK, TX	1301 Young Street Dallas, TX 75202	(214) 767-3301
Region 7: IA, KS, MO, NE	Bolling Federal Building 601 East 12th Street Kansas City, MO 64106	(816) 426-2821
Region 8: CO, MT, ND, SD,UT, WY	Bryon G. Rogers Federal Office Building 1961 Stout Street Room 1076 Denver, CO 80294	(303) 844-3372
Region 9: AZ, CA, HI, NV, American Samoa, Guam, Commonwealth of the Northern Mariana Islands, Federated States of Micronesia, Republic of the Marshall Islands, Republic of Palau	Federal Office Building 50 United Nations Plaza San Francisco, CA 94102	(415) 437-8500
Region 10: AK, ID, OR, WA	Blanchard Plaza Bldg. 2201 6th Avenue Seattle, WA 98121	(206) 615-2010

Source: U.S. Department of Health and Human Services. HHS Region Map. Available at http://www.hhs.gov/about/regionmap.html. Accessed October 6, 2010.

of the Assistant Secretary for Preparedness and Response (ASPR) now constitute the Public Health Service (PHS). Another three operating divisions (CMS, ACF, and AoA) comprise the human services operating divisions.

Administration on Aging (AoA)

This division of the HHS is the principal agency designated to carry out the provisions of the Older Americans Act of 1965. This agency
tracks the characteristics, circumstances, and needs of older people; develops policies, plans, and programs to promote their welfare; administers grant programs to benefit older Americans; and administers training, research, demonstration programs, and protective services for older Americans. One exemplary program supported by the AoA is Meals on Wheels.

Administration for Children and Families (ACF)
The ACF is composed of a number of smaller agencies and is responsible for providing direction and leadership for all federal programs for needy children and families. One of the better-known programs originating from this division is Head Start, which serves more than 900,000 preschool children. Other programs are aimed at family assistance, refugee resettlement, and child support enforcement.

Agency for Healthcare Research and Quality (AHRQ)
Prior to 1999, this division of the HHS was called the Agency for Health Care Policy and Research, but its name was changed as part of the Healthcare Research and Quality Act of 1999. AHRQ is "the Nation's lead Federal agency for research on health care quality, costs, outcomes, and patient safety."[12] AHRQ sponsors and conducts research that provides evidence-based information on health care outcomes; quality; and cost, use, and access. The information helps health care decision makers—patients and clinicians, health system leaders, and policy makers—make more informed decisions and improve the quality of health care services.

Agency for Toxic Substances and Disease Registry (ATSDR)
This agency was created by the **Superfund legislation** (Comprehensive Environmental Response, Compensation, and Liability Act) in 1980. This legislation was enacted to deal with the cleanup of hazardous substances in the environment. ATSDR's mission is to "serve the public through responsive public health actions to promote healthy and safe environments and prevent harmful exposures."[13] To carry out its mission and to serve the needs of the American public, ATSDR evaluates information on hazardous substances released into the environment in order to assess the impact on public health; conducts and sponsors studies and other research related to hazardous substances and adverse human health effects; establishes and maintains registries of human exposure (for long-term follow-up) and complete listings of areas closed to the public or otherwise restricted in use due to contamination; summarizes and makes data available on the effects of hazardous substances; and provides consultations and training to ensure adequate response to public health emergencies. Although ATSDR has been responding to chemical emergencies in local communities across the country for the last 25 years, like many of the other federal health agencies its work has taken on new meaning since 9/11. For example, some of the projects the agency's staff have worked on or continue to work on include sampling dust in New York City residences after 9/11; working with New York health agencies to create a registry of people who lived or worked near the World Trade Center (WTC) on 9/11 to collect health information on those most heavily exposed to smoke, dust, and debris from the collapse of the WTC; conducting environmental sampling at anthrax-contaminated buildings; and disseminating critical information to agencies and organizations with a role in terrorism preparedness and response.[14]

Superfund legislation
legislation enacted to deal with the cleanup of hazardous substances in the environment

Centers for Disease Control and Prevention (CDC)
The CDC, located in Atlanta, Georgia (see Figure 3), "is the nation's premiere health promotion, prevention, and preparedness agency and global leader in public health."[15] The CDC serves as the national focus for developing and applying disease prevention (including bioterrorism) and control, environmental health, and health promotion and education activities designed to improve the health of the people of the United States.[15] Once known solely for its work to control communicable diseases, the CDC now also maintains records, analyzes disease trends, and publishes epidemiological reports on all types of diseases, including those that result from lifestyle, occupational, and environmental causes. Beyond its own specific responsibilities, the CDC also supports state and local health departments and cooperates with similar national health agencies from other WHO member nations.

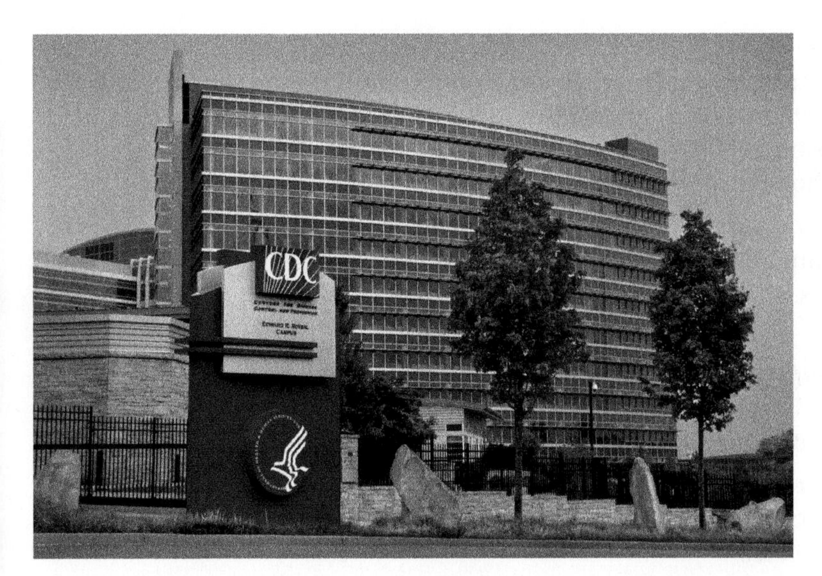

FIGURE 3
The Centers for Disease Control and Prevention (CDC) in Atlanta, Georgia, is one of the major operating agencies of the Department of Health and Human Services.

To better meet the challenges of public health for the twenty-first century, in 2003, the CDC began a strategic planning process called the *Futures Initiative.*[15] As a part of the Futures Initiative, the CDC adopted new overarching health protection goals and a new organizational structure. The goals that were adopted included the following:

- *Preparedness:* People in all communities will be protected from infectious, environmental, and terrorist threats.
- *Health promotion and prevention of disease, injury, and disability:* All people will achieve their optimal life span with the best possible quality of health in every stage of life.
- *Healthy places:* The places where people live, work, learn, and play should protect and promote human health and eliminate health disparities.

The reorganization of the CDC, as a result of the Futures Initiative, created a structure that included the Office of the Director, the National Institute for Occupational Safety and Health (NIOSH), and six coordinating centers/offices. More recently, the CDC engaged in ongoing reorganization that changed the organizational structure of the agency. The CDC's Centers, Institutes, and Offices (CIOs) "allow the agency to be more responsive and effective when dealing with public health concerns. Each group implements the CDC's response in their areas of expertise, while also providing intra-agency support and resource-sharing for cross-cutting issues and specific health threats."[15] The CIOs, as of June 2010, include the following:

- *Center for Global Health:* Includes the Division of Global HIV/AIDS, Division of Parasitic Diseases and Malaria, Division of Global Disease Detection and Emergency Response, and the Division of Public Health Systems and Workforce Development
- *National Institute for Occupational Safety and Health (NIOSH):* Includes the Health Effects Laboratory Division; Education and Information Division; Division of Applied Research and Technology; Division of Respiratory Disease Studies; Division of Safety Research; Division of Surveillance, Hazard Evaluations and Field Studies; the National Personal Protective Technology Laboratory; the Office of Mine Safety and Health; and the Division of Compensation, Analysis and Support
- *Office of Infectious Diseases:* Includes the Influenza Coordination Unit; the National Center for Immunization and Respiratory Diseases; the National Center for HIV/AIDS, Viral Hepatitis, STD and TB Prevention; and the National Center for Emerging and Zoonotic Infectious Diseases
- *National Center for Immunization and Respiratory Diseases (NCIRD):* Includes the Influenza Division, Division of Viral Diseases, Division of Bacterial Diseases, Global Immunizations Division, and the Immunization Services Division
- *National Center for Emerging and Zoonotic Infectious Diseases (NCEZID):* (In 2010, NCEZID was a new center in transition; therefore, the following was updated April

2010.) Includes the Food Safety Office; the Division of Foodborne, Waterborne, and Environmental Diseases; the Division of Preparedness and Emerging Infections; the Division of Global Migration and Quarantine; the Division of Scientific Resources; the Division of Healthcare Quality Promotion; the Division of Vector-Borne Diseases; and the Division of High-Consequence Pathogens and Pathology

- *National Center for HIV/AIDS, Viral Hepatitis, STD, and TB Prevention (NCHHSTP):* Includes the Division of Sexually Transmitted Diseases Prevention, Division of HIV/AIDS Prevention, the Division of Viral Hepatitis, the Division of Tuberculosis Elimination, the Global AIDS Program (GAP)
- *Office of Noncommunicable Diseases, Injury and Environmental Health:* Includes the Division of Environmental Hazards and Health Effects, the Division of Emergency and Environmental Health Services, and the Division of Laboratory Sciences
- *National Center on Birth Defects and Developmental Disabilities:* Includes the Division of Human Development and Disability, the Division of Blood Disorders, and the Division of Birth Defects and Developmental Disabilities
- *National Center for Chronic Disease Prevention and Health Promotion:* Includes the Division of Adolescent and School Health; the Division of Adult and Community Health; the Division of Cancer Prevention and Control; the Division of Diabetes Translation; the Division of Nutrition, Physical Activity and Obesity; the Division of Oral Health; the Division of Reproductive Health; the Office on Smoking and Health; and the Division for Heart Disease and Stroke Prevention
- *National Center for Environmental Health/Agency for Toxic Substances and Disease Registry:* Includes the Division for Emergency and Environmental Health Services, the Division of Environmental Hazards and Health Effects, the Division of Laboratory Sciences, the Division of Health Assessment and Consultation, the Division of Health Studies, the Division of Regional Operations, and the Division of Toxicology and Environmental Medicine
- *National Center for Injury Prevention and Control:* Includes the Division of Injury Response, the Division of Unintentional Injury Prevention, and the Division of Violence Prevention
- *Office of Public Health Preparedness and Response:* Includes the Division of Emergency Operations, the Division of State and Local Readiness, the Division of Strategic National Stockpile, and the Division of Select Agents and Toxins
- *Office for State, Trial, Local and Territorial Support:* Includes the Division of Public Health Performance Improvement and the Division of Public Health Capacity Development
- *Office of Surveillance, Epidemiology, and Laboratory Services (OSELS is proposed for agency approval, as of June 2010, and will include the following, if approved):* Includes the National Center for Health Statistics; the National Office of Public Health Genomics; the Laboratory Science, Policy and Practice Program Office; the Public Health Informatics and Technology Program Office; the Public Health Surveillance Program Office; the Epidemiology and Analysis Program Office; and the Scientific Education and Professional Development Program Office
- *National Center for Health Statistics:* Includes the Classifications and Public Health Data Standards Staff, the Division of Health Examination Statistics, the Division of Health Care Surveys, the Division of Health Interview Statistics, the Division of Vital Statistics, the Office of Analysis and Epidemiology, and the Office of Research and Methodology[15]

Food and Drug Administration (FDA)

The FDA touches the lives of virtually every American every day. It "is charged with protecting the public health by ensuring the safety, efficacy, and security of human and veterinary drugs, biological products, and medical devices; ensuring the safety of foods, cosmetics, and radiation-emitting products; and regulating tobacco products.

Specifically, FDA is responsible for advancing the public health by:

- Helping to speed innovations that make medicines and foods safer and more effective
- Providing the public with the accurate, science-based information they need to use medicines and foods to improve their health
- Regulating the manufacture, marketing, and distribution of tobacco products to protect the public and reduce tobacco use by minors
- Addressing the nation's counterterrorism capability and ensuring the security of the supply of foods and medical products."[16]

Much of this work revolves around regulatory activities and the setting of health and safety standards as spelled out in the Federal Food, Drug, and Cosmetic Act and other related laws. However, because of the complex nature of its standards and the agency's limited resources, enforcement of many FDA regulations is left to other federal agencies and to state and local agencies. For example, the Department of Agriculture is responsible for the inspection of many foods, such as meat and dairy products. Restaurants, supermarkets, and other food outlets are inspected by state and local public health agencies.

Centers for Medicare and Medicaid Services (CMS)

Established as the Health Care Financing Administration (HFCA) in 1977, the CMS is responsible for overseeing the Medicare program (health care for the elderly and the disabled), the federal portion of the Medicaid program (health care for low-income individuals), and the related quality assurance activities. Both Medicare and Medicaid were created in 1965 to ensure that the special groups covered by these programs would not be deprived of health care because of cost. In 2008, about 99 million Americans were covered by these programs.[9] In 1997, the Children's Health Insurance Program (CHIP) also became the responsibility of the CMS.

Health Resources and Services Administration (HRSA)

The HRSA is the principal primary health care service agency of the federal government that provides access to essential health care services for people who are low-income, uninsured, or who live in rural areas or urban neighborhoods where health care is scarce.[9] It "is the primary federal agency for improving access to health care services for people who are underinsured, isolated, or medically vulnerable."[17] The cited mission of HRSA is "to improve health and achieve health equity through access to quality services, a skilled health workforce and innovative programs."[17] HRSA "maintains the National Health Service Corps and helps build the health care workforce through training and education programs."[9] The agency "administers a variety of programs to improve the health of mothers and children and serves people living with HIV/AIDS through the Ryan White CARE Act programs."[9] HRSA is also responsible for overseeing the nation's organ transplantation system.[9]

Indian Health Service (IHS)

The IHS "is responsible for providing federal health services to American Indians and Alaska Natives."[18] Currently, it "provides a comprehensive health service delivery system for approximately 1.9 million American Indians and Alaska Natives who belong to 564 federally recognized tribes in 35 states."[18] "The provision of health services to members of federally recognized tribes grew out of the special government-to-government relationship between the federal government and Indian tribes. This relationship, established in 1787, is based on Article I, Section 8 of the Constitution, and has been given form and substance by numerous treaties, laws, Supreme Court decisions, and Executive Orders. The IHS is the principal federal health care provider and health advocate for Indian people."[18] The mission of the IHS is "to raise the physical, mental, social, and spiritual health of American Indians and Alaska Natives to the highest level,"[18] while its goal is "to assure that comprehensive, culturally acceptable personal and public health services are available and accessible to American Indian and Alaska Native people."[18]

Though health services have been provided sporadically by the United States government since the early nineteenth century, it was not until 1989 that the IHS was elevated to an agency level; prior to that time it was a division in HRSA.

National Institutes of Health (NIH)

Begun as a one-room Laboratory of Hygiene in 1887, the NIH today is one of the world's foremost medical research centers, and the federal focal point for medical research in the United States.[19] The mission of the NIH "is to seek fundamental knowledge about the nature and behavior of living systems and the application of that knowledge to enhance health, lengthen life, and reduce the burdens of illness and disability."[19] Although a significant amount of research is carried out by NIH scientists at NIH laboratories in Bethesda and elsewhere, a much larger portion of this research is conducted by scientists at public and private universities and other research institutions. These scientists receive NIH funding for their research proposals through a competitive, peer-review grant application process. Through this process of proposal review by qualified scientists, NIH seeks to ensure that federal research monies are spent on the best-conceived research projects. Table 3 provides a listing of all the institutes and centers located in NIH.

Table 3
Units within the National Institutes of Health (NIH)

National Cancer Institute (NCI)
National Eye Institute (NEI)
National Heart, Lung, and Blood Institute (NHLBI)
National Human Genome Research Institute (NHGRI)
National Institute on Aging (NIA)
National Institute on Alcohol Abuse and Alcoholism (NIAAA)
National Institute of Allergy and Infectious Diseases (NIAID)
National Institute of Arthritis and Musculoskeletal and Skin Diseases (NIAMS)
National Institute of Biomedical Imaging and Bioengineering (NIBIB)
Eunice Kennedy Shriver National Institute of Child Health and Human Development (NICHD)
National Institute on Deafness and Other Communication Disorders (NIDCD)
National Institute of Dental and Craniofacial Research (NIDCR)
National Institute of Diabetes and Digestive and Kidney Diseases (NIDDK)
National Institute on Drug Abuse (NIDA)
National Institute of Environmental Health Sciences (NIEHS)
National Institute of General Medical Sciences (NIGMS)
National Institute of Mental Health (NIMH)
National Institute of Neurological Disorders and Stroke (NINDS)
National Institute of Nursing Research (NINR)
National Library of Medicine (NLM)
NIH Clinical Center (CC)
Center for Information Technology (CIT)
National Center for Complementary and Alternative Medicine (NCCAM)
National Center on Minority Health and Health Disparities (NCMHD)
National Center for Research Resources (NCRR)
John E. Fogarty International Center for Advanced Study in the Health Sciences (FIC)
Center for Scientific Review (CSR)

Source: National Institutes of Health (2010). "Institutes, Centers and Offices." Available at http://www.nih.gov/icd/. Accessed October 6, 2010.

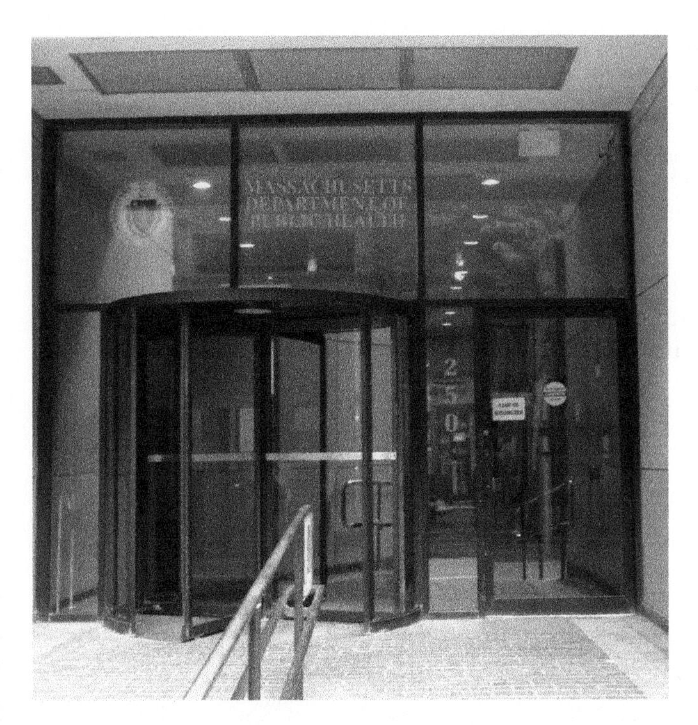

FIGURE 4
Each of the 50 states has its own health department.

Substance Abuse and Mental Health Services Administration (SAMHSA)
The SAMHSA is the primary federal agency responsible for ensuring that up-to-date information and state-of-the-art practice are effectively used for the prevention and treatment of addictive and mental disorders. "SAMHSA's mission is to reduce the impact of substance abuse and mental illness on American's communities."[20] Within SAMHSA, there are three centers—the Center for Substance Abuse Treatment (CSAT), the Center for Substance Abuse Prevention (CSAP), and the Center for Mental Health Services (CMHS). Additionally, the agency houses one office, the Office of Applied Studies (OAS), which is responsible for "the collection, analysis and dissemination of behavioral health data."[20] Each of these centers has its own mission that contributes to the overall mission of SAMHSA.

State Health Agencies

All 50 states have their own state health departments (see Figure 4). Although the names of these departments may vary from state to state (e.g., Ohio Department of Health, Indiana State Department of Health), their purposes remain the same: to promote, protect, and maintain the health and welfare of their citizens. These purposes are represented in the **core functions of public health**, which include *assessment* of information on the health of the community, comprehensive public health *policy development,* and *assurance* that public health services are provided to the community.[21] These core functions have been defined further with the following 10 essential public health services.[22]

core functions of public health assessment, policy development, and assurance

1. Monitor health status to identify community health problems.
2. Diagnose and investigate health problems and health hazards in the community.
3. Inform, educate, and empower people about health issues.
4. Mobilize community partnerships to identify and solve health problems.
5. Develop policies and plans that support individual and community health efforts.
6. Enforce laws and regulations that protect health and ensure safety.
7. Link people to needed personal health services and assure the provision of health care when otherwise unavailable.
8. Ensure a competent public health and personal health care workforce.
9. Evaluate effectiveness, accessibility, and quality of personal- and population-based health services.
10. Research for new insights and innovative solutions to health problems (see Figure 5).

The head of the state health department is usually a medical doctor, appointed by the governor, who may carry the title of director, commissioner, or secretary. However, because of the political nature of the appointment, this individual may or may not have extensive experience in community or public health. Unfortunately, political influence sometimes reaches below the level of commissioner to the assistant commissioners and division chiefs; it is the commissioner, assistant commissioners, and division chiefs who set policy and provide direction for the state health department. Middle- and lower-level employees are usually hired through a merit system and may or may not be able to influence health department policy. These employees, who carry out the routine work of the state health department, are usually professionally trained health specialists such as microbiologists, engineers, sanitarians, epidemiologists, nurses, and health education specialist.

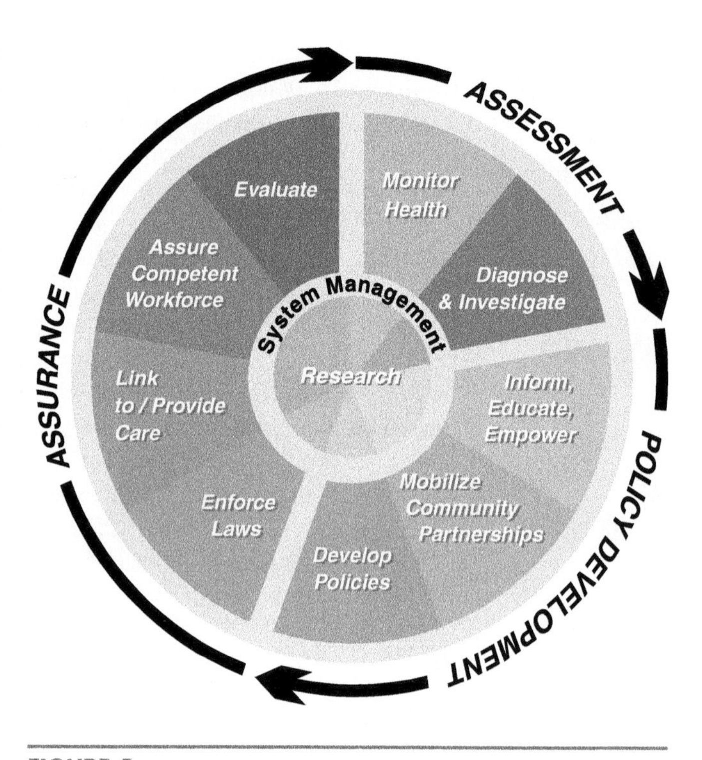

FIGURE 5

Core functions of public health and the 10 essential services.

Source: Public Health Functions Steering Committee, Members (July 1995). "Public Health in America." Available at http://web.health.gov/phfunctions/public.htm. Accessed October 28, 2010.

Most state health departments are organized into divisions or bureaus that provide certain standard services. Typical divisions include Administration, Communicable Disease Prevention and Control, Chronic Disease Prevention and Control, Vital and Health Statistics, Environmental Health, Health Education or Promotion, Health Services, Maternal and Child Health, Mental Health, Occupational and Industrial Health, Dental Health, Laboratory Services, Public Health Nursing, Veterinary Public Health, and most recently, a division of Public Health Preparedness to deal with bioterrorism issues.

In promoting, protecting, and maintaining the health and welfare of their citizens, state health departments play many different roles. They can establish and promulgate health regulations that have the force and effect of law throughout the state. The state health departments also provide an essential link between federal and local (city and county) public health agencies. As such, they serve as conduits for federal funds aimed at local health problems. Federal funds come to the states as block grants. Funds earmarked for particular health projects are distributed to local health departments by their respective state health departments in accordance with previously agreed upon priorities. State health departments may also link local needs with federal expertise. For example, epidemiologists from the CDC are sometimes made available to investigate local disease outbreaks at the request of the state health department. State health departments usually must approve appointments of local health officers and can also remove any local health officers who neglect their duties.

The resources and expertise of the state health department are also at the disposal of local health departments. One particular area where the state health departments can be helpful is laboratory services; many modern diagnostic tests are simply too expensive for local health departments. Another area is environmental health. Water and air pollution problems usually extend beyond local jurisdictions, and their detection and measurement often require equipment too expensive for local governments to afford. This equipment and expertise are often provided by the state health department.

Local Health Departments

Local-level governmental health organizations, referred to as local health departments (LHDs), are usually the responsibility of the city or county governments. In large metropolitan areas, community health needs are usually best served by a city health department. In smaller cities with populations of up to 75,000, people often come under the jurisdiction of a county health department. In some rural counties where most of the population is concentrated in a single city, a LHD may have jurisdiction over both city and county residents. In sparsely populated rural areas, it is not uncommon to find more than one county served by a single health department. In 2008, there were approximately 2,794 LHDs; of that number, 64% were located in nonmetropolitan areas and 36% were in metropolitan areas.[23]

It is through LHDs that health services are provided to the people of the community. A great many of these services are mandated by state laws, which also set standards for health and safety. Examples of mandated local health services include the inspection of restaurants, public buildings, and public transportation systems; the detection and reporting of certain diseases; and the collection of vital statistics such as births and deaths. Other programs such as safety belt programs and immunization clinics may be locally planned and implemented. In this regard, local health jurisdictions are permitted (unless preemptive legislation is in place) to enact ordinances that are stricter than those of the state, but these jurisdictions cannot enact codes that fall below state standards. It is at this level of governmental health agencies that sanitarians implement the environmental health programs, nurses and physicians offer the clinical services, and health education specialists present health education and promotion programs.

Organization of Local Health Departments

Each LHD is headed by a health officer/administrator/commissioner (see Figure 6). In most states, there are laws that prescribe who can hold such a position. Those often noted are physicians, dentists, veterinarians, or individuals with a master's or doctoral degree in public health. If the health officer is not a physician, then a physician is usually hired on a consulting basis to advise as needed. Usually, this health officer is appointed by a board of health, the members of which are themselves appointed by officials in the city or county government or, in some situations, elected by the general public. The health officer and administrative assistants may recommend which programs will be offered by the LHDs. However, they may need final approval from a board of health. Although it is desirable that those serving on the local board of health have some knowledge of community health programs, most states have no such requirement. Often, politics plays a role in deciding the makeup of the local board of health.

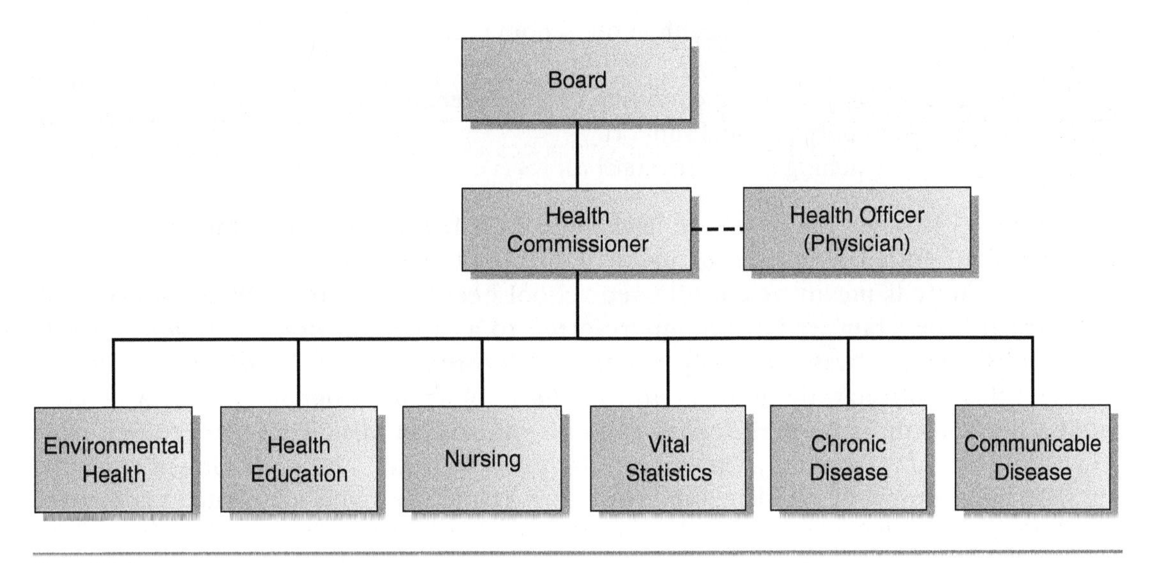

FIGURE 6
Organizational chart of a local public health agency.

The local health officer, like the state health commissioner, has far-reaching powers, including the power to arrest someone who refuses to undergo treatment for a communicable disease (tuberculosis, for example) and who thereby continues to spread disease in the community. The local health officer has the power to close a restaurant on the spot if it has serious health law violations or to impound a shipment of food if it is contaminated. Because many local health departments cannot afford to employ a full-time physician, the health officer is usually hired on a part-time basis. In such cases, the day-to-day activities of the LHD are carried out by an administrator trained in public health. The administrator is also hired by the board of health based upon qualifications and the recommendation of the health officer.

Local sources provide the greatest percentage of LHD revenues (25%), followed by state funds (20%) and federal pass-through funds (17%).[23] A limited number of LHD services are provided on a fee-for-service basis. For example, there is usually a fee charged for birth and death certificates issued by the LHD. Also, in some communities, minimal fees are charged to offset the cost of providing immunizations, lab work, or inspections. Seldom do these fees cover the actual cost of the services provided. Therefore, income from service fees usually makes up a very small portion of any LHD budget. And, it is not unusual to find that many LHDs use a **sliding scale** to determine the fee for a service.

sliding scale the scale used to determine the fee for services based on ability to pay

Coordinated School Health Programs

Few people think of public schools as governmental health agencies. Consider, however, that schools are funded by tax dollars, are under the supervision of an elected school board, and include as a part of their mission the improvement of the health of those in the school community. Because school attendance is required throughout the United States, the potential for school health programs to make a significant contribution to community health is enormous. In fact, Allensworth and Kolbe have stated that schools "could do more perhaps than any other single agency in society to help young people, and the adults they will become, to live healthier, longer, more satisfying, and more productive lives."[24] Yet coordinated school health programs have faced a number of barriers, including the following:[25]

1. Insufficient local administrative commitment
2. Inadequately prepared teachers
3. Too few school days to teach health in the school year
4. Inadequate funding
5. The lack of credibility of health education as an academic subject
6. Insufficient community/parental support
7. Concern for the teaching of controversial topics (i.e., sex education)

If communities were willing to work to overcome these barriers, the contribution of coordinated school health programs to community health could be almost unlimited.

What exactly is meant by coordinated school health? Prior to 1998, a coordinated school health program was commonly referred to as a *comprehensive school health program*. However, it was commonly confused with *comprehensive health education*. To eliminate this confusion, the term *coordinated* school health program is used. A coordinated school health program is defined as "an organized set of policies, procedures, and activities designed to protect, promote, and improve the health and well-being of students and staff, thus improving a student's ability to learn. It includes but is not limited to comprehensive school health education; school health services; a healthy school environment; school counseling; pyschological and social services; physical education; school nutrition services; family and community involvement in school health; and school-site health promotion for staff."[28]

Though all components of the coordinated school health program are important, there are three essential components: health education, a healthy school environment, and health services. Health instruction should be based on a well-conceived, carefully planned curriculum that has an appropriate scope (coverage of topics) and logical sequencing. Instructional units should include cognitive (knowledge), affective (attitudes), and psychomotor (behavioral) components. The healthy school environment should provide a learning environment that is both physically and mentally safe and healthy. Finally, each school's health program should provide the essential health services, from emergency care through health appraisals, to ensure that students will be healthy learners.

Quasi-Governmental Health Organizations

quasi-governmental health organizations organizations that have some responsibilities assigned by the government but operate more like voluntary agencies

The **quasi-governmental health organizations**—organizations that have some official health responsibilities but operate, in part, like voluntary health organizations—make important contributions to community health. Although they derive some of their funding and legitimacy from governments, and carry out tasks that may be normally thought of as government work, they operate independently of government supervision. In some cases, they also receive financial support from private sources. Examples of quasi-governmental agencies are the American Red Cross (ARC), the National Science Foundation, and the National Academy of Sciences.

The American Red Cross

The ARC, founded in 1881 by Clara Barton (see Figure 7), is a prime example of an organization that has quasi-governmental status. Although it has certain "official" responsibilities placed on it by the federal government, it is funded by voluntary contributions. "Official" duties of the ARC include (1) providing relief to victims of natural disasters such as floods, tornadoes, hurricanes, and fires (Disaster Services) and (2) serving as the liaison between members of the active armed forces and their families during emergencies (Services to the Armed Forces and Veterans). In this latter capacity, the ARC can assist active-duty members of the armed services in contacting their families in case of an emergency, or vice versa.

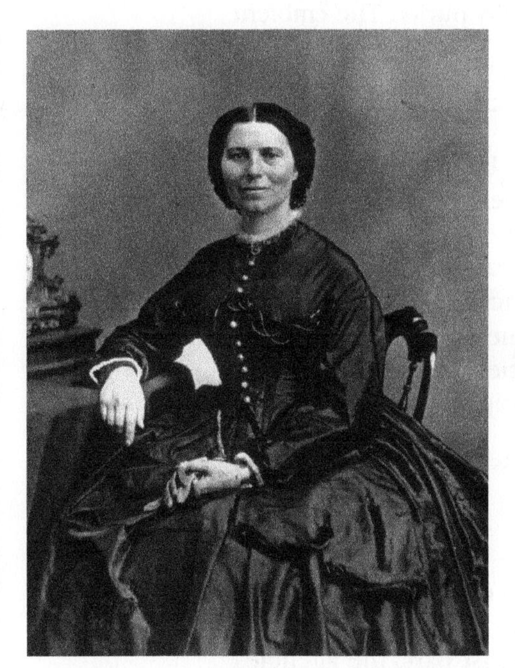

FIGURE 7
The American Red Cross was founded by Clara Barton in 1881.

In addition to these "official" duties, the ARC also engages in many nongovernmental services. These include blood drives, safety services (including water safety, first aid, CPR, and HIV/AIDS instruction), nursing and health services, youth services, community volunteer services, and international services.

The ARC was granted a charter by Congress in 1900, and the ARC and the federal government have had a special relationship ever since. The president of the United States is the honorary chairman of the ARC. The U.S. Attorney General and Secretary of the Treasury are honorary counselor and treasurer, respectively.

The Red Cross idea was not begun in the United States. It was begun in 1863 by five Swiss men in Geneva, Switzerland, who were concerned with the treatment provided to the wounded during times of war. The group, which was called the International Committee for the Relief to the Wounded, was led by Henry Dunant. With the assistance of the Swiss government, the International Committee brought together delegates from 16 nations in 1864 to the Geneva Convention for the Amelioration of the Condition of the Wounded in Armies in the Field (now known as the first Geneva Convention) to sign the Geneva Treaty.

The efforts of Henry Dunant and the rest of the International Committee led to the eventual establishment of the International Committee of the Red Cross (ICRC). The ICRC, which still has its headquarters in Geneva and is still governed by the Swiss, continues to work today during times of disaster and international conflict. It is the organization that visits prisoners of war to ensure they are being treated humanely.[29,30]

Content removed due to copyright restrictions

Today, the international movement of the Red Cross comprises the Geneva-based ICRC, the International Federation of Red Cross and Red Crescent Societies (the red crescent emblem is used in Moslem countries), and the over 180 National Red Cross and Red Crescent Societies.[29] There are a number of other countries that believe in the principles of the Red Cross Movement, but have not officially joined because the emblems used by the movement are offensive. Thus, the ICRC has created a third emblem that meets all the criteria for use as a protective device and at the same time is free of any national, political, or religious connotations. The design is composed of a red frame in the shape of a square on the edge of a white background. The name chosen for this distinctive emblem was "red crystal," to signify purity. The emblem was put into use on January 14, 2007 (see Figure 8).[30]

Other Quasi-Governmental Organizations

Two other examples of quasi-governmental organizations in the United States are the National Science Foundation (NSF) and the National Academy of Sciences (NAS). The purpose of NSF is the funding and promotion of scientific research and the development of individual scientists. NSF receives and disperses federal funds but operates independently of governmental supervision. Chartered by Congress in 1863, the NAS acts as an advisor to the government on questions of science and technology. Included in its membership are some of America's most renowned scientists. Although neither of these agencies exists specifically to address health problems, both organizations fund projects, publish reports, and take public stands on health-related issues.

Nongovernmental Health Agencies

Nongovernmental health agencies are funded by private donations or, in some cases, by membership dues. There are thousands of these organizations that all have one thing in common: They arose because there was an unmet need. For the most part, the agencies operate free from governmental interference as long as they meet Internal Revenue Service guidelines with regard to their specific tax status. In the following sections, we discuss the following types of nongovernmental health agencies—voluntary, professional, philanthropic, service, social, religious, and corporate.

Voluntary Health Agencies

voluntary health agencies
nonprofit organizations created by concerned citizens to deal with a health need not met by governmental health agencies

Voluntary health agencies are an American creation. Each of these agencies was created by one or more concerned citizens who felt that a specific health need was not being met by existing governmental agencies. In a sense, these new voluntary agencies arose by themselves, in much the same way as a "volunteer" tomato plant arises in a vegetable garden. New voluntary agencies continue to be born each year. Examples of recent additions to the perhaps 100,000 agencies already in existence are the Alzheimer's Association and the First Candle (formerly SIDS Alliance). A discussion of the commonalities of voluntary health agencies follows.

Organization of Voluntary Health Agencies

Most voluntary agencies exist at three levels—national, state, and local. At the national level, policies that guide the agency are formulated. A significant portion of the money raised locally is forwarded to the national office, where it is allocated according to the agency's budget. Much of the money is designated for research. By funding research, the agencies hope to discover the cause of and cure for a particular disease or health problem. There have been some major successes. The March of Dimes, for example, helped to eliminate polio as a major disease problem in the United States through its funding of immunization research.

There is not always a consensus of opinion about budget decisions made at the national level; some believe that less should be spent for research and more for treating those afflicted with the disease. Another common internal disagreement concerns how much of the funds raised at the local level should be sent to the national headquarters instead of being retained for local use. Those outside the agency sometimes complain that when an agency achieves success, as the March of Dimes did in its fight against polio, it should dissolve. This does not usually occur; instead, successful agencies often find a new health concern. The March of Dimes now fights birth defects; and when tuberculosis was under control, the Tuberculosis Society changed its name to the American Lung Association to fight all lung diseases.

The state-level offices of voluntary agencies are analogous to the state departments of health in the way that they link the national headquarters with local offices. The primary work at this level is to coordinate local efforts and to ensure that policies developed at the national headquarters are carried out. The state-level office may also provide training services for employees and volunteers of local-level offices and are usually available as consultants and problem solvers. In recent years, some voluntary agencies have been merging several state offices into one to help reduce overhead expenses.

The local-level office of each voluntary agency is usually managed by a paid staff worker who has been hired either by the state-level office or by a local board of directors. Members of the local board of directors usually serve in that capacity on a voluntary basis. Working under the manager of each agency are local volunteers, who are the backbone of voluntary agencies. It has been said that the local level is where the "rubber meets the road." In other words, this is where most of the money is raised, most of the education takes place, and most of the service is rendered. Volunteers are of two types, professional and lay. Professional volunteers have had training in a medical profession, while lay volunteers have had no medical training. The paid employees help facilitate the work of the volunteers with expertise, training, and other resources.

Purpose of Voluntary Health Agencies

Voluntary agencies share four basic objectives: (1) to raise money to fund their programs, with the majority of the money going to fund research, (2) to provide education both to professionals and to the public, (3) to provide service to those individuals and families that are afflicted with the disease or health problem, and (4) to advocate for beneficial policies, laws, and regulations that affect the work of the agency and in turn the people they are trying to help.

Fund-raising is a primary activity of many voluntary agencies. Whereas in the past this was accomplished primarily by door-to-door solicitations, today mass-mailing and telephone solicitation are more common. In addition, most agencies sponsor special events such as golf outings, dances, or dinners. One type of special event that is very popular today is the "a-thon" (see Figure 9). The term "a-thon" is derived from the name of the ancient Greek city Marathon and usually signified some kind of "endurance" event. Examples include bike-a-thons, rock-a-thons, telethons, skate-a-thons, and dance-a-thons. These money-making "a-thons" seem to be limited in scope only by the creativity of those planning them. In addition, some of these agencies have become United Way agencies and receive some funds derived from the annual United Way campaign, which conducts fund-raising efforts at worksites. The three largest voluntary agencies in the United States today (in terms of dollars raised) are the American Cancer Society (see Box 1), the American Heart Association, and the American Lung Association.

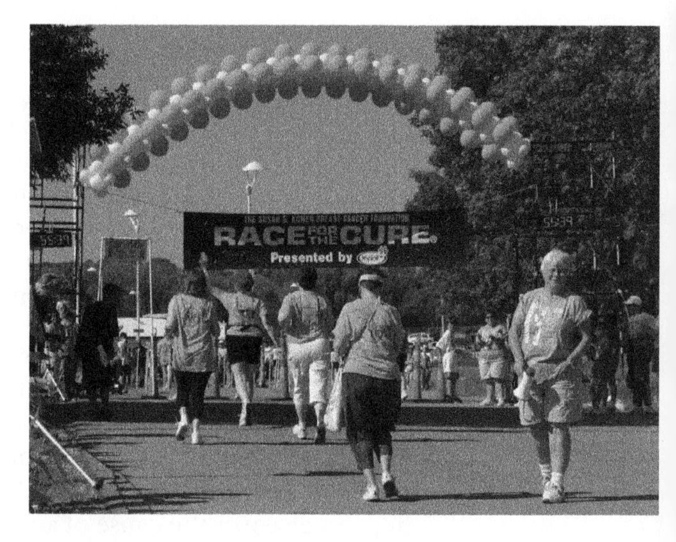

FIGURE 9
Most voluntary health agencies hold special events to raise money for their causes.

Over the years, the number of voluntary agencies formed to help meet special health needs has continually increased. Because of the growth in the number of new agencies, several consumer "watchdog" groups have taken a closer look into the practices of the agencies. A major concern of these consumer groups has been the amount of money that the voluntary agencies spend on the cause (e.g., cancer, heart disease, AIDS) and how much they spend on fund-raising and overhead (e.g., salaries, office furniture, leasing of office space). Well-run agencies will spend less than 15% of what they raise on fund-raising. Some of the not-so-well-run agencies spend as much as 80% to 90% on fund-raising. All consumers should ask agencies how they spend their money prior to contributing.

Professional Health Organizations/Associations

Professional health organizations and associations are made up of health professionals who have completed specialized education and training programs and have met the standards of registration, certification, and/or licensure for their respective fields. Their mission is to promote high standards of professional practice for their specific profession, thereby improving the health of society by improving the people in the profession. Professional organizations are funded primarily by membership dues. Examples of such organizations are the American Medical Association, the American Dental Association, the American Nursing Association, the American Public Health Association, the American Association for Health Education, and the Society for Public Health Education, Inc.

Although each professional organization is unique, most provide similar services to their members. These services include the certification of continuing-education programs for professional renewal, the hosting of annual conventions where members share research results and interact with colleagues, and the publication of professional journals and other reports. Some examples of journals published by professional health associations are the *Journal of the American Medical Association,* the *American Journal of Public Health,* and the *American Journal of Health Education.*

BOX 1

A Closer Look at One Voluntary Health Agency: The American Cancer Society

The American Cancer Society (ACS) was founded in 1913 by 10 physicians and 5 laymen. At that time, it was known as the American Society for the Control of Cancer. Today, with offices throughout the country and approximately 2 million volunteers, ACS is one of our largest voluntary health organizations. In spite of its success, its mission has remained constant since its founding. It is "dedicated to eliminating cancer as a major health problem by preventing cancer, saving lives, and diminishing suffering from cancer, through research, education, advocacy and service."[31]

The mission of the ACS includes both short- and long-term goals. Its short-term goals are to save lives and diminish suffering. This is accomplished through education, advocacy, and service. Its long-term goal, the elimination of cancer, is being approached through the society's support of cancer research.

The American Cancer Society's educational programs are targeted at two different groups—the general public and the health professionals who treat cancer patients. The public education program promotes the following skills and concepts to people of all ages: (1) taking the necessary steps to prevent cancer, (2) knowing the seven warning signals, (3) understanding the value of regular checkups, and (4) coping with cancer. The society accomplishes this by offering free public education programs, supported by up-to-date literature and audiovisual materials, whenever and wherever they may be requested. These programs may be presented in homes, worksites, churches, clubs, organizations, and schools. A few of their better-known programs include I Can Cope, Reach to Recovery, and Man to Man.[31] From time to time, the society also prepares public service messages for broadcasting or televising.

The society's professional education program is aimed at the professionals who work with oncology patients. The objective of this program is to motivate physicians and other health care professionals "to maintain and improve their knowledge of cancer prevention, detection, diagnosis, treatment, and palliative care."[32] Such education is provided through professional publications, up-to-date audiovisual materials, conferences, and grants that fund specialized education experiences.

The ACS offers patient service and rehabilitation programs that ease the impact of cancer on those affected. The services offered include information and referral to appropriate professionals, home care supplies and equipment for the comfort of patients, transportation of patients to maintain their medical and continuing care programs, and specialized education programs for cancer patients to help them cope and feel better about themselves. There are also rehabilitation programs that provide social support for all cancer patients and specific programs for those who have had a mastectomy, laryngectomy, or ostomy.

The ACS is the largest source of private, not-for-profit cancer research funds in the United States, second only to the federal government in total dollars spent. Since 1946, when the ACS first started awarding grants, it has invested about $3.1 billion in cancer research. The research program consists of three components: extramural grants, intramural epidemiology and surveillance research, and the intramural behavioral research center.[31] The most recent addition to the work of the ACS is in the area of advocacy. Specifically, the ACS works to (1) support cancer research and programs to prevent, detect, and treat cancer; (2) expand access to quality cancer care, prevention, and awareness; (3) reduce cancer disparities in minority and medically underserved populations; and (4) reduce and prevent suffering from tobacco-related illnesses.[31]

All ACS programs—education, service, research, and advocacy—are planned primarily by the society's volunteers. However, the society does employ staff members to carry out the day-to-day operations and to help advise and support the work of the volunteers. This arrangement of volunteers and staff working together has created a very strong voluntary health agency.

Like voluntary health agencies, another important activity of some professional organizations is advocating on issues important to their membership. The American Medical Association, for example, has a powerful lobby nationally and in some state legislatures. Their purpose is to affect legislation in such a way as to benefit their membership and their profession. Many professional health organizations provide the opportunity for benefits, including group insurance and discount travel rates. There are hundreds of professional health organizations in the United States, and it would be difficult to describe them all here.

philanthropic foundation an endowed institution that donates money for the good of humankind

Philanthropic Foundations

Philanthropic foundations have made and continue to make significant contributions to community health in the United States and throughout the world. These foundations support community health by funding programs and research on the prevention, control, and treatment of many diseases. Foundation directors, sometimes in consultation with a review committee, determine the types of programs that will be funded. Some foundations fund an array of health projects, whereas others have a much narrower scope of interests. Some foundations, such as the Bill and Melinda Gates Foundation, fund international health projects, whereas others restrict their funding to domestic projects. The geographical scope of domestic foundations can be national, state, or local. Local foundations may restrict their funding to projects that only benefit local citizens.

The activities of these foundations differ from those of the voluntary health agencies in two important ways. First, foundations have money to give away, and therefore no effort is spent on fund-raising. Second, foundations can afford to fund long-term or innovative research projects, which might be too risky or expensive for voluntary or even government-funded agencies. The development of a vaccine for yellow fever by a scientist funded by the Rockefeller Foundation is an example of one such long-range project.

Some of the larger foundations, in addition to the Bill and Melinda Gates Foundation, that have made significant commitments to community health are the Commonwealth Fund, which has contributed to community health in rural communities, improved hospital facilities, and tried to strengthen mental health services; the Ford Foundation, which has contributed greatly to family-planning efforts throughout the world; the Robert Wood Johnson Foundation, which has worked to improve access to medical and dental care throughout the United States and lessen the impact of tobacco on health; the Henry J. Kaiser Family Foundation, which has supported the development of health maintenance organizations (HMOs) and community health promotion; the W. K. Kellogg Foundation, which has funded many diverse health programs that address human issues and provide a practical solution; and the Milbank Memorial Fund, which has primarily funded preventive-medicine projects.

Service, Social, and Religious Organizations

Service, social, and religious organizations have also played a part in community health over the years (see Figure 10). Examples of service and social groups involved in community health are the Jaycees, Kiwanis Club, Fraternal Order of Police, Rotary Club, Elks, Lions, Moose, Shriners, American Legion, and Veterans of Foreign Wars. Members of these groups enjoy social interactions with people of similar interests in addition to fulfilling the groups' primary reason for existence—service to others in their communities. Although health may not

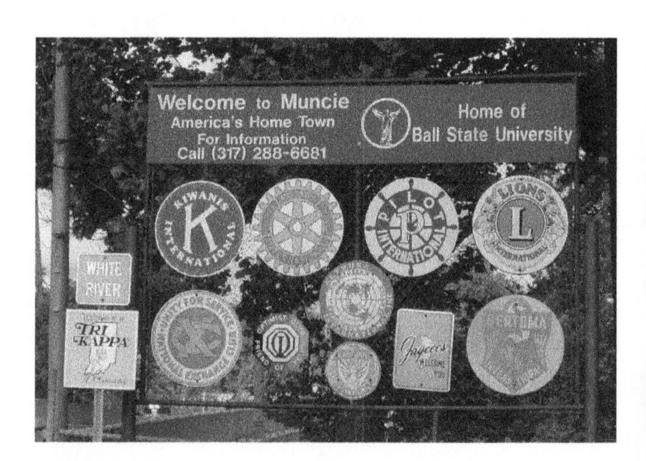

FIGURE 10
Community service groups contribute needed resources for the improvement of the health of the community.

be the specific focus of their mission, several of these groups make important contributions in that direction by raising money and funding health-related programs. Sometimes, their contributions are substantial. Examples of such programs include the Shriners' children's hospitals and burn centers; the Lions' contributions to pilot (lead) dog programs and other services for those who are visually impaired, such as the provision of eyeglasses for school-aged children unable to afford them; and the Lions' contributions to school health programs via the educational program named "Lions Quest."

The contributions of religious groups to community health have also been substantial. Such groups also have been effective avenues for promoting health programs because (1) they have had a history of volunteerism and preexisting reinforcement contingencies for volunteerism, (2) they can influence entire families, and (3) they have accessible meeting-room facilities.[33] One way in which these groups contribute is through donations of money for missions for the less fortunate. Examples of religious organizations that solicit donations from their members include the Protestants' One Great Hour of Sharing, the Catholics' Relief Fund, and the United Jewish Appeal. Other types of involvement in community health by religious groups include (1) the donation of space for voluntary health programs such as blood donations, Alcoholics Anonymous, and other support groups, (2) the sponsorship of food banks and shelters for the hungry, poor, and homeless, (3) the sharing of the doctrine of good personal health behavior, and (4) allowing community health professionals to deliver their programs through the congregations. This latter contribution has been especially useful in black American communities because of the importance of churches in the culture of this group of people.

In addition, it should be noted that some religious groups have hindered the work of community health workers. Almost every community in the country can provide an example where a religious organization has protested the offering of a school district's sex education program, picketed a public health clinic for providing reproductive information or services to women, or has spoken out against homosexuality.

Corporate Involvement in Community Health

From the way it treats the environment by its use of natural resources and the discharge of wastes, to the safety of the work environment, to the products and services it produces and provides, to the provision of health care benefits for its employees, corporate America is very much involved in community health. Though each of these aspects of community health is important to the overall health of a community, because of the concern for the "bottom line" in corporate America, it is the provision of health care benefits that often receives the most attention. In fact, many corporations today find that their single largest annual expenditure behind salaries and wages is for employee health care benefits. Consider, for example, the cost of manufacturing a new car. The cost of health benefits for those who build the car now exceeds the cost of the raw materials for the car itself.

In an effort to keep a healthy workforce and reduce the amount paid for health care benefits, many companies support health-related programs both at and away from the worksite. Worksite programs aimed at trimming employee medical bills have been expanded beyond the traditional safety awareness programs and first aid services to include such programs as substance abuse counseling, nutrition education, smoking cessation, stress management, physical fitness, and disease management. Many companies also are implementing health promotion policies and enforcing state and local laws that prohibit (or severely restrict) smoking on company grounds or that mandate the use of safety belts at all times in all company-owned vehicles.

Chapter Summary

- Contemporary society is too complex to respond effectively to community health problems on either an emergency or a long-term basis. This fact necessitates organizations and planning for health in our communities.
- The different types of organizations that contribute to the promotion, protection, and maintenance of health in a community can be classified into three groups according to their sources of funding and organizational structure—governmental, quasi-governmental, and nongovernmental.
- Governmental health agencies exist at the local, state, federal, and international levels and are funded primarily by tax dollars.
- WHO is the largest and most visible governmental health agency on the international level.
- The Department of Health and Human Services (HHS) is the U.S. government's principal agency for the protection of the health of all Americans and for providing essential human services, especially for those who are least able to help themselves.
- The core functions of public health include the assessment of information on the health of the community, comprehensive public health policy development, and assurance that public health services are provided to the community.
- Quasi-governmental agencies, such as the American Red Cross, share attributes with both governmental and nongovernmental agencies.
- Nongovernmental organizations include voluntary and professional associations, philanthropic foundations, and service, social, and religious groups.
- Corporate America has also become more involved in community health, both at the worksite and within the community.

Review Questions

1. What characteristics of modern society necessitate planning and organization for community health?
2. What is a governmental health agency?
3. What is the World Health Organization (WHO), and what does it do?
4. What federal department in the United States is the government's principal agency for protecting the health of all Americans and for providing essential human services, especially to those who are least able to help themselves? What major services does this department provide?
5. What are the three core functions of public health?
6. What are the 10 essential public health services?
7. How do state and local health departments interface?
8. What is meant by the term *coordinated school health program*? What are the major components of it?
9. What is meant by the term *quasi-governmental agency*? Name one such agency.
10. Describe the characteristics of a nongovernmental health agency.
11. What are the major differences between a governmental health organization and a voluntary health agency?
12. What does a health professional gain from being a member of a professional health organization?
13. How do philanthropic foundations contribute to community health? List three well-known foundations.

Scenario: Analysis and Response

After having read this chapter, please respond to the following questions in reference to the scenario at the beginning of the chapter.

1. What type of health agency do you think will be of most help to Mary?
2. If this scenario were to happen to someone in your community, what recommendations would you give to him or her on seeking help from health agencies?
3. The Internet has many sources of information that could help Mary. Use a search engine (e.g., Google) and enter the word "cancer." Find the Web site of one governmental health agency at the national level and one voluntary health agency that might be able to help her. Explain how these agencies could be of help.
4. If Mary did not have Internet access, how would you suggest she find out about local health agencies in her area that could help her?

14. How do service, social, and religious groups contribute to the health of the community?
15. Why has corporate America become involved in community health?

Activities

1. Using a local telephone book, list all the health-related organizations that service your community. Divide your list by the three major types of health organizations noted in this chapter.
2. Make an appointment to interview someone at one of the organizations identified in Activity 1. During your visit, find answers to the following questions:
   a. How did the organization begin?
   b. What is its mission?
   c. How is it funded?
   d. How many people (employees and volunteers) work for the organization, and what type of education/training do they have?
   e. What types of programs/services does the organization provide?
3. Obtain organizational charts from the U.S. Department of Health and Human Services (a copy is in this chapter), your state department of health, and your local health department. Compare and contrast these charts, and describe their similarities and differences.
4. Call a local voluntary health organization in your community and ask if you could volunteer to work 10 to 15 hours during this academic term. Then, volunteer those hours and keep a journal of your experience.
5. Carefully review your community newspaper each day for an entire week. Keep track of all articles or advertisements that make reference to local health organizations. Summarize your findings in a one-page paper. (If you do not subscribe to your local paper, copies are available in libraries.)

Community Health on the Web

The Internet contains a wealth of information about community and public health. Increase your knowledge of some of the topics presented in this chapter by accessing the Jones & Bartlett Learning Web site at **http://health.jbpub.com/book/communityhealth/7e** and follow the links to complete the following Web activities.

- World Health Organization
- Department of Health and Human Services
- Association of State and Territorial Health Officials

References

1. Green, L. W. (1990). "The Revival of Community and the Public Obligation of Academic Health Centers." In R. E. Bulger and S. J. Reiser, eds., *Integrity in Institutions: Humane Environments for Teaching, Inquiry and Health*. Iowa City: University of Iowa Press, 163–180.
2. World Health Organization (2010). "World Health Organization." Available at http://www.who.int/about/en/.
3. World Health Organization (2003). *World Health Report 2003: Shaping the Future*. Geneva, Switzerland: Author.
4. United Nations (2000). *United Nations Millennium Declaration*. New York: Author.
5. United Nations (2002). *Road Map Towards the Implementation of the United Nations Millennium Declaration*. New York: Author.
6. United Nations (2007). *The Millennium Development Goals Report*. New York: Author.
7. Dodd, R., and A. Cassels (2006). "Health, Development and the Millennium Development Goals." *Annals of Tropical Medicine and Parasitology*, 100(5/6): 379–387.
8. World Health Organization (2005). *Health and the Millennium Development Goals*. Geneva, Switzerland: Author.
9. U.S. Department of Health and Human Services (2010). "United States Department of Health and Human Services." Available at http://www.hhs.gov/about/whatwedo.html.
10. Government Printing Office Access (2010). *Budget of the United States Government: Browse Fiscal Year 2010*. Available at http://origin.www.gpoaccess.gov/usbudget/fy10/browse.html.
11. U.S. Department of Health and Human Services (2010). "Health Reform and the Department of Human Services." Available at http://www.healthreform.gov/health_reform_and_hhs.html.
12. Agency for Healthcare Research and Quality (2010). "What Is AHRQ?" Available at http://www.ahrq.gov/about/Whatis.htm.
13. Agency for Toxic Substances and Disease Registry (2006). "About the Agency for Toxic Substances and Disease Registry." Available at http://www.atsdr.cdc.gov/about.index.html.
14. Falk, H. (2003) "A Message from Dr. Henry Falk, ATSDR Assistant Administrator." *Public Health and the Environment*, 2(1/2): 1.
15. Centers for Disease Control and Prevention (2010). "Centers for Disease Control and Prevention." Available at http://www.cdc.gov/.
16. U.S. Food and Drug Administration (2010). "Strategic Priorities 2011–2015: Responding to the Public Health Challenges of the 21st Century, DRAFT 9/29/2010." Available at http://www.fda.gov/AboutFDA/ReportsManualsForms/Reports/ucm227527.htm#mission.
17. Health Resources and Services Administration (2006). "About HRSA." Available at http://www.hrsa.gov/about/default.htm.
18. Indian Health Service (2010). "Indian Health Service Introduction." Available at http://www.ihs.gov/PublicInfo/PublicAffairs/Welcome_Info/IHSintro.asp.
19. National Institutes for Health (2010). "Questions and Answers about NIH." Available at http://www.nih.gov/about/mission.htm.
20. Substance Abuse and Mental Health Services Administration (2010). "SAMSHA: Who Are We?" Available at http://www.samhsa.gov/about/background.aspx.
21. National Academy of Sciences, Institute of Medicine (1988). *The Future of Public Health*. Washington, DC: National Academy Press.
22. Office of Disease Prevention and Health Promotion (2008). "Public Health in America." Available at http://web.health.gov/phfunctions/public.htm.
23. National Association of County and City Health Officials (2009). *2008 National Profile of Local Health Departments*. Washington, DC: Author.
24. Allensworth, D. D., and L. J. Kolbe (1987). "The Comprehensive School Health Program: Exploring an Expanded Concept." *Journal of School Health*, 57(10): 409–412.

25. Butler, S. C. (1993). "Chief State School Officers Rank Barriers to Implementing Comprehensive School Health Education." *Journal of School Health*, 63(3): 130–132.

26. Clark, N. M. (2002). *A Letter from the Dean*. Ann Arbor, MI: University of Michigan, School of Public Health.

27. Institute of Medicine (2003). *The Future of the Public's Health*. Washington, DC: National Academies Press.

28. Joint Committee on Health Education and Promotion Terminology (2001). "Report of the 2000 Joint Committee on Health Education and Promotion Terminology." *American Journal of Health Education*, 32(2): 89–103.

29. American Red Cross (2010). "Red Cross History." Available at http://www.redcross.org/.

30. International Committee of the Red Cross (2006). "About the International Committee of the Red Cross—ICRC." Available at http://www.icrc.org.

31. American Cancer Society (2006). "About the American Cancer Society." Available at http://www.cancer.org/docroot/AA/AA_0.asp.

32. American Cancer Society (2006). "Continuing Medical Education." Available at http://www.cancer.org/docroot/PRO/content/PRO_2_Continuing_Medical_Education.asp.

33. Lasater, T. M., B. L. Wells, R. A. Carleton, and J. P. Elder (1986). "The Role of Churches in Disease Prevention Research Studies." *Public Health Report*, 101(2): 123–131.

PHOTO CREDITS

3 Courtesy of James Gathany/CDC; **7** © National Library of Medicine; **9** © Suzanne Tucker/ShutterStock, Inc.

Unless otherwise indicated, all photographs and illustrations are under copyright of Jones & Bartlett Learning, or have been provided by the authors.

Community Organizing/ Building and Health Promotion Programming

Chapter Outline

Chapter Objectives

After studying this chapter, you will be able to:

1. Define *community organizing, community capacity, community participation,* and *empowered community.*
2. Identify the assumptions that underlie the process of community organization.
3. Briefly explain the difference between locality development, social planning, and social action approaches to community organization.
4. Explain the difference between needs-based and strength-based community organizing models.
5. List the steps for a generalized model for community organizing/building.
6. Explain what is meant by community building.
7. Explain the difference between health education and health promotion.
8. State and summarize the steps involved in creating a health promotion program.
9. Define the term *needs assessment.*
10. Briefly explain the six steps used in assessing needs.
11. Explain the difference between goals and objectives.
12. List the different types of intervention strategies.
13. Explain the differences among best practices, best experiences, and best processes.
14. Explain the purposes of pilot testing in program development.
15. State the difference between formative and summative evaluation.

SCENARIO

It was becoming obvious to many that the suburb of Kenzington now had a drug problem, but few wanted to admit it. The community's residents liked their quiet neighborhoods, and most never thought that drugs would be a problem. In fact, the problem really sneaked up on everyone. The town had only one bar, and although occasionally someone drank too much, the bar's patrons usually controlled their drinking and didn't bother anyone. Occasionally, two or three high school seniors would be caught drinking beer purchased at a store in a nearby town. Yet these isolated incidents gave no indication of Kenzington's impending drug problem.

Within the past year, the climate of the town had changed considerably. Incidents of teenagers being arrested for possession of alcohol or even other drugs, such as marijuana, were being reported more regularly in the newspaper. There seemed to be more reports of burglaries, too. There had even been a robbery and two assaults reported within the last month. The population of young adults in the community seemed to be increasing, and many of these seemed to be driving impressive cars, using the hottest new digital devices, and wearing the latest clothes. All of these signs were obvious to a group of concerned citizens in Kenzington and suggested the possibility of a drug problem. So the concerned citizens decided to take their concern to the city council.

INTRODUCTION

To deal with the health issues that face many communities, community health professionals must possess specific knowledge and skills. They need to be able to identify problems, develop a plan to attack each problem, gather the resources necessary to carry out that plan, implement that plan, and then evaluate the results to determine the degree of progress that has been achieved. In the previous two chapters, we described epidemiological methods as essential tools of the community health professional. In this chapter, we present two other important tools that each successful community health worker must master: the skills to organize/build a community and to plan a health promotion program. Prior to presenting information about community organizing/building and health promotion programming, we need to introduce the concept of *social ecological approach*.

Inherent in the community organizing/building and health promotion programming processes is behavior change. That is, for community organizing/building and health promotion programming efforts to be successful people must change their behavior. Some of the behaviors that need to change as part of these processes are health-related and others are not. The underlying foundation of the social ecological approach is that behavior has multiple levels of influences. This approach "emphasizes the interaction between, and the interdependence of factors within and across all levels of a health problem"[1] That is to say, seldom does behavior change based on influence from a single level. People "live in social, political, and economic systems that shape behaviors and access to the resources they need to maintain good health."[2] Scholars who study and write about the levels of influence have used various labels to describe them. However, commonly used labels include intrapersonal, interpersonal, institutional or organizational, community, and public policy.[3] These five levels are presented in a hierarchical order with the first level, intrapersonal, affecting a single person, with successive levels affecting greater numbers, and the highest level—public policy—affecting the most. For example, to get a person to participate in a community coalition it may take someone to talk with the person (e.g., intrapersonal-level influence) about the importance of the work of the coalition, but it might also take the organization with which the person is affiliated to include the work of the coalition in its mission statement (i.e., organizational-level influence). Or, to get a person to stop smoking it may take a conversation with his/her physician (i.e., intrapersonal-level influence), a company policy (i.e., institutional- or organizational-level), and also a county ordinance prohibiting smoking in public places (i.e., community-level influence). Thus, a central conclusion of the social ecological approach "is that it usually takes the combination of both individual-level and environmental/policy-level interventions to achieve substantial changes in health behavior."[4]

As you read the rest of this chapter, consider the impact of the social ecological approach on both community/organizing and health promotion programming.

Community Organizing/Building

Community health problems can range from small and simple to large and complex. Small, simple problems that are local and involve few people can be solved with the effort of a small group of people and a minimal amount of organization. Large, complex problems that involve whole communities require significant skills and resources for their solution. For these larger problems, a considerable effort must be expended to organize the citizens of the community to work together to implement a lasting solution to their problem. For example, a trained smoking cessation facilitator could help a single person or a small group of people to stop smoking. But to reduce the smoking rates community-wide, community collaboration is needed. The same smoking cessation facilitators are needed to work with individuals, but others are also needed. Schools are needed to provide appropriate tobacco education programs to youth, organizations (e.g., worksites) and institutions (e.g., religious communities) are needed to create smoking policies, government agencies are needed to enforce the laws associated with the sale of tobacco, and cities, counties, and states are needed to create clean indoor air ordinances or laws. This more comprehensive approach to reducing smoking rates needs to bring together, in an organized and coordinated effort, the people and groups interested in the issue and the resources necessary for change. In other words, a community organization effort is needed.

community organizing process through which communities are helped to identify common problems or goals, mobilize resources, and in other ways develop and implement strategies for reaching their goals they have collectively set

"The term *community organization* was coined by American social workers in the late 1880s to describe their efforts to coordinate services for newly arrived immigrants and the poor."[5] More recently, *community organization* has been used by a variety of professionals, including community health workers, and refers to various methods of interventions to deal with social problems. More formally, **community organizing** has been defined as a "process through which communities are helped to identify common problems or goals, mobilize resources, and in other ways develop and implement strategies for reaching their goals they have collectively set."[5] Community organizing is not a science but an art of consensus building within a democratic process.[6] (See Table 1 for terms associated with community organizing/building).

Table 1
Terms Associated with Community Organizing/Building

Term	Definition
Community capacity	"The characteristics of communities that affect their ability to identify, mobilize, and address social and public health problems"[7]
Empowerment	"Social action process for people to gain mastery over their lives and the lives of their communities"[8]
Participation and relevance	"Community organizing that starts where the people are and engages community members as equals"[5]
Social capital	"Relationships and structures within a community that promote cooperation for mutual benefit"[5]

Need for Organizing Communities

In recent years, the need to organize communities seems to have increased. Advances in electronics (e.g., handheld digital devices) and communications (e.g., multifunction cell phones and the Internet), household upgrades (e.g., energy efficiency), and increased mobility (i.e., frequency of moving and ease of worldwide travel) have resulted in a loss of a sense of community. Individuals are much more independent than ever before. The days when people knew everyone on their block are past. Today, it is not uncommon for people to never meet their neighbors (see Figure 1). In other cases, people see or talk to their neighbors only once or twice each year. Because of these changes in community social structure, it now takes specific skills to organize a community to act together for the collective good. Note that the usefulness of community organizing skills extends beyond community health.

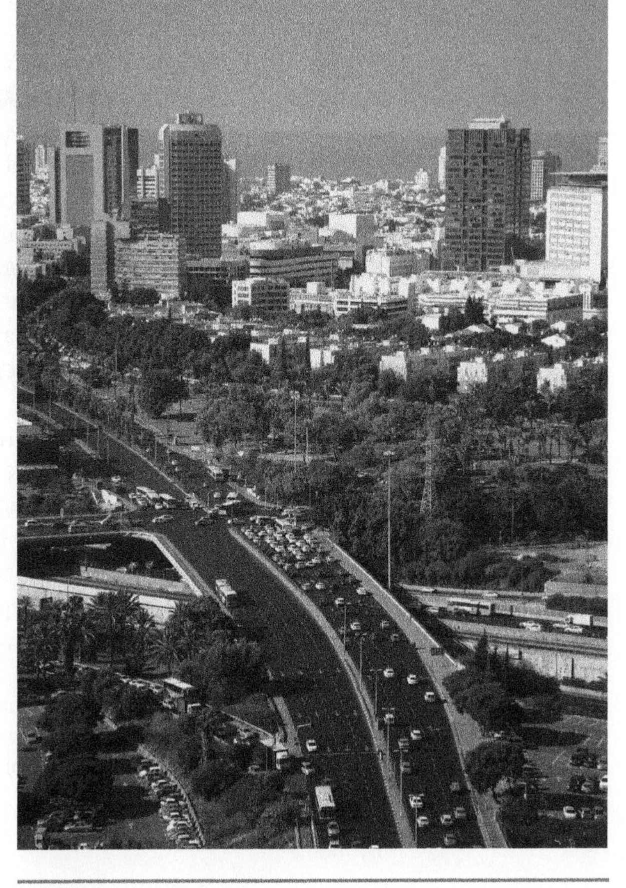

FIGURE 1
In today's complex communities, it is not uncommon for people never to meet their neighbors.

Assumptions of Community Organizing

According to Ross,[6] those who organize communities do so while making certain assumptions. The assumptions Ross outlines can be summarized as follows:

1. Communities of people can develop the capacity to deal with their own problems.
2. People want to change and can change.
3. People should participate in making, adjusting, or controlling the major changes taking place within their communities.
4. Changes in community living that are self-imposed or self-developed have a meaning and permanence that imposed changes do not have.
5. A "holistic approach" can successfully address problems with which a "fragmented approach" cannot cope.
6. Democracy requires cooperative participation and action in the affairs of the community, and people must learn the skills that make this possible.
7. Frequently, communities of people need help in organizing to deal with their needs, just as many individuals require help in coping with their individual problems.

Community Organizing Methods

There is no single, preferred method for organizing a community. In fact, a careful review reveals that several different approaches have been successful, which led Rothman and Tropman to state, "We would speak of community organization methods rather than the community organization method."[9]

The early approaches to community organization used by social workers emphasized the use of consensus and cooperation to deal with community problems.[10] However, Rothman created a typology of three primary methods of community organization.[11] Included were locality development, social planning, and social action.[9] *Locality development* is based on the concept of broad self-help participation from the local community. It is "heavily process oriented, stressing consensus and cooperation aimed at building group identity and a sense of community."[5]

Social planning is heavily task oriented, stressing rational-empirical problem solving and involves various levels of participation from many people and outside planners.[5]

The third method, *social action,* is "both task and process oriented"[5] and has been useful in helping to organize disadvantaged segments of the population. It often involves trying to redistribute power or resources, which enables institutional or community change. This method is not used as much as it once was, but it was useful during the civil rights and gay rights movements and in other settings where people have been oppressed.

Though locality development, social planning, and social action methods have been the primary means by which communities have organized over the years, they do have their limitations. Maybe the greatest limitation is that they are primarily "problem-based and organizer-centered, rather than strength-based and community-centered."[12] Thus, some of the newer models are based more on collaborative empowerment and community building. However, all models—old or new—revolve around a common theme: The work and resources of many have a much better chance of solving a problem than the work and resources of a few.

Minkler and Wallerstein have done a nice job of summarizing the models, old and new, by presenting a typology that incorporates both needs- and strength-based approaches (see Figure 2).[5] Their typology is divided into four quadrants, with strength-based and needs-based on the vertical axis and consensus and conflict on the horizontal axis. Though this typology separates and categorizes the various methods of community organizing and building, Minkler and Wallerstein point out that

> Community organizing and community building are fluid endeavors. While some organizing efforts primarily have focused in one quadrant, most incorporate multiple tendencies, possibly starting from a specific need or crisis and moving to a strength-based community capacity

approach. Different organizing models, such as coalitions, lay health worker programs, political action groups, leadership development or grassroots organizing may incorporate needs- or strength-based approaches at different times, depending on the starting place and the ever changing social dynamic. It is important, however, that organizing efforts clarify their assumptions and make decisions about primary strategies based on skills of group members, history of the group, willingness to take risks, or comfort level with different approaches.[5]

No matter what community organizing/community building approach is used, they all incorporate some fundamental principles. These include "the principle of relevance, or starting where the people are; the principle of participation; and the importance of creating environments in which individuals and communities can become empowered as they increase their community problem-solving ability."[5]

Content removed due to copyright restrictions

The Process of Community Organizing/Building

It is beyond the scope of this textbook to explain all the approaches to community organizing and building in detail. Instead, we will present a generic approach (see Figure 3) created by McKenzie, Neiger, and Thackeray that draws upon many of these other approaches.[13] The 10 steps of this generic approach are briefly reviewed in the sections that follow.

Recognizing the Issue

The process of community organizing/building begins when someone recognizes that a problem exists in a community and decides to do something about it. This person (or persons) is referred to as the initial organizer. This individual may not be the primary organizer throughout the community organizing/building process. He or she is the one who gets things started. For the purposes of this discussion, let us assume the problem is violence. People in most communities would like to have a violence-free community, but it would be most unusual to live in a community that was without at least some level of violence. How much violence is too much? At what point is a community willing to organize to deal with the problem? In a small-town community, an acceptable level of violence would be very low, while in a large city, an acceptable level would be much higher.

The people, or organizers, who first recognize a problem in the community and decide to act can be members of the community or individuals from outside the community. If those who initiate community organization are members of the community, then the movement is

grass-roots
a process that begins with those who are affected by the problem/concern

referred to as being **grass-roots**, *citizen initiated,* or organized from the *bottom up*. "In *grassroots organizing*, community groups are built from scratch, and leadership is developed where none existed before."[14] Community members who might recognize that violence is a problem could include teachers, police officers, or other concerned citizens. When community organization is initiated by individuals from outside of the community, the problem is said to be organized from the *top down* or *outside in.* Individuals from outside the community who might initiate organization could include a judge who presides over cases involving violence, a state social worker who handles cases of family violence, or a politically active group that is against violent behavior wherever it happens. In cases where the person who recognizes the community problem is not a community member, great care must be taken when notifying those in the community that a problem exists. "It is difficult for someone from the outside coming in and telling community members that they have problems or issues that have to be dealt with and they need to organize to take care of them."[13]

Gaining Entry into the Community

This second step in the community organizing process may or may not be needed, depending on whether the issue in step 1 was identified by someone from within the community or outside. If the issue is identified by someone outside the community, this step becomes a critical step in the process.[13] Gaining entry may seem like a relatively easy matter, but an error by organizers at this step could ruin the chances of successfully organizing the community. This may be the most crucial step in the whole process.

gatekeepers
those who control, both formally and informally, the political climate of the community

Braithwaite and colleagues have stressed the importance of tactfully negotiating entry into a community with the individuals who control, both formally and informally, the "political climate" of the community.[15] These people are referred to as the **gatekeepers**. Thus the term indicates that you must pass through this "gate" to get to your priority population.[16] These "power brokers" know their community, how it functions, and how to accomplish tasks within it. Long-time residents are usually able to identify the gatekeepers of their community. A gatekeeper can be a representative of an intermediary organization—such as a church or school—that has direct contact with your priority population.[16] Examples include politicians, leaders of activist groups, business and education leaders, and clergy, to name a few.

Organizers must approach such figures on the gatekeepers' own terms and play the gatekeepers' ball game. However, before approaching these important individuals, organizers must study the community well. They must be *culturally sensitive* and work toward *cultural competence*. That is, they must be aware of the cultural differences within a community and effectively work with the cultural context of the community. Tervalon and Garcia have stated the need for *cultural humility*—openness to others' culture.[17] Organizers need to know where the power lies, the community power dynamics, what type of politics must be used to solve a problem, and whether the particular problem they wish to solve has ever been dealt with before in the community.[18] In the violence example, organizers need to know (1) who is causing the violence and why, (2) how the problem has been addressed in the past, (3) who supports and who opposes the idea of addressing the problem, and (4) who could provide more insight into the problem. This is a critical step in the community organization process because failure to study the community carefully in the beginning may lead to a delay in organizing it later, a subsequent waste of time and resources, and possibly the inability to organize at all.

Once the organizers have a good understanding of the community, they are then ready to approach the gatekeepers. In keeping with the violence example, the gatekeepers would probably include the police department, elected officials, school board members, social service personnel, members of the judicial system, and possibly some of those who are creating the violence.

When the top-down approach is being used, organizers might find it advantageous to enter the community through a well-respected organization or institution that is already established in the community, such as a church, a service group, or another successful local group. If those who make up such an organization/institution can be convinced that the problem exists and needs to be solved, it can help smooth the way for gaining entry and achieving the remaining steps in the process.

Organizing the People

Obtaining the support of community members to deal with the problem is the next step in the process. It is best to begin by organizing those who are already interested in seeing that the problem is solved. This core group of community members, sometimes referred to as "executive participants,"[19] will become the backbone of the workforce and will end up doing the majority of the work. For our example of community violence, the core group could include law enforcement personnel, former victims of violence and their families (or victims' support groups), parent-teacher organizations, and public health officials. It is also important to recruit people from the subpopulation that is most directly affected by the problem. For example, if most of the violence in a community is directed toward teenagers, teenagers need to be included in the core group. If elderly persons are affected, they need to be included.

"From among the core group, a leader or coordinator must be identified. If at all possible, the leader should be someone with leadership skills, good knowledge of the concern and the community, and most of all, someone from within the community. One of the early tasks of the leader will be to help build group cohesion."[13]

Although the formation of the core group is essential, this group is usually not large enough to do all the work itself. Therefore, one of the core group's tasks is to recruit more members of the community to the cause. This step can take place via a *networking process,* which is when organizers make personal contacts with others who might be interested. Or, the organizers can call an organizing meeting at a local school, community center, or religious organization. By broadening the constituency, the core group can spread out the workload and generate additional resources to deal with the problem. However, recruiting additional workers can often be difficult. Over the last 30 years, the number of people in many communities interested in volunteering their time has decreased. Today, if you ask someone to volunteer, you may hear the reply, "I'm already too busy." There are two primary reasons for this response. First, there are many families in which both husband and wife work outside the home. And second, there are more single-parent households.

Therefore, when organizers are expanding their constituencies, they should be sure to (1) identify people who are affected by the problem that they are trying to solve, (2) provide "perks" for or otherwise reward volunteers, (3) keep volunteer time short, (4) match volunteer assignments with the abilities and expertise of the volunteers, and (5) consider providing appropriate training to make sure volunteers are comfortable with their tasks. For example, if the organizers need someone to talk with law enforcement groups, it would probably be a good idea to solicit the help of someone who feels comfortable around such groups and who is respected by them, such as another law enforcement person.

task force
a temporary group that is brought together for dealing with a specific problem

coalition
formal alliance of organizations that come together to work for a common goal

When the core group has been expanded to include these other volunteers, the larger group is sometimes referred to as a task force. A **task force** has been defined as "a self-contained group of 'doers' that is not ongoing, but rather brought together due to a strong interest in an issue and for a specific purpose."[14] There may even be an occasion where a coalition is formed. A **coalition** is "a formal alliance of organizations that come together to

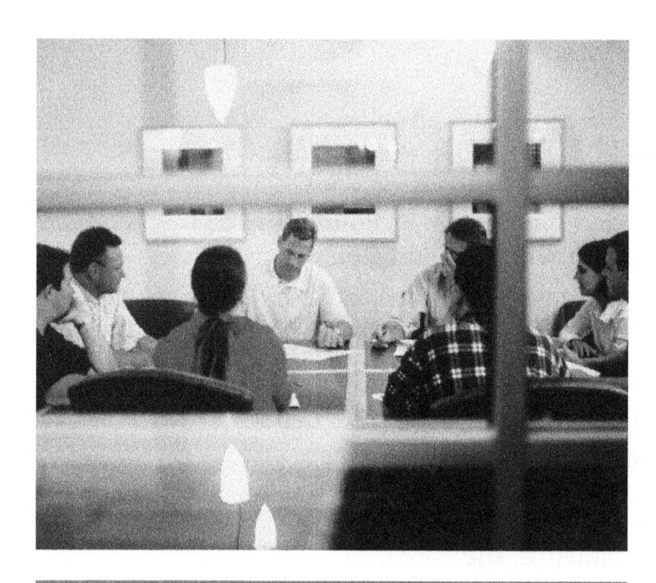

FIGURE 4
Coalition building is often an important step in successful community organization.

work for a common goal"[14]—often, to compensate for deficits in power, resources, and expertise. A larger group with more resources, people, and energy has a greater chance of solving a community problem than a smaller, less powerful group (see Figure 4). "Building and maintaining effective coalitions have increasingly been recognized as vital components of much effective community organizing and community building."[20]

Assessing the Community

Earlier in this chapter we referred to Rothman and Tropman's typology for organizing a community—locality development, social planning, and social action.[9] Each of these community organizing strategies operates "from the assumption that problems in society can be addressed by the community becoming better or differently 'organized,' with each strategy perceiving the problems and how or whom to organize in order to address them somewhat differently."[15] In contrast to these strategies is community building. **Community building** "is an orientation to community that is strength-based rather than need-based and stresses the identification, nurturing, and celebration of community assets."[21] Thus, one of the major differences between community organizing and community building is the type of assessment that is used to determine where to focus the community's efforts. In the community organizing approach, the assessment is focused on the needs of the community, while in community building, the assessment focuses on the assets and capabilities of the community. It is assumed that a clearer picture of the community will be revealed and a stronger base will be developed for change if the assessment includes the identification of both needs and assets/capacities and involves those who live in the community. It is from these capacities and assets that communities are built.[22]

community building
an orientation to community that is strength-based rather than need-based and stresses the identification, nurturing, and celebration of community assets

To determine the needs and assets/capacities of a community, an assessment must be completed. There are two reasons for completing an effective and comprehensive assessment: "Information is needed for change, and it is also needed for empowerment."[23] This could include a traditional *needs assessment* and/or a newer technique called *mapping community capacity*. A needs assessment is a process by which data about the issues of concern are collected and analyzed. From the analyzed data, concerns or problems emerge and are prioritized so that strategies can be created to tackle them.

Traditional forms of data collection for needs assessments have included techniques such as completing written questionnaires or interviewing people in the community. Because of the importance of getting participation from community members and "starting where the people are,"[24] some organizers have used *participatory data collection* processes. Such processes get those from whom the data are to be collected to help with data collection. One newer technique for doing this is call *photovoice*.[25,26] With this technique community members are provided with cameras and skills training, and then they use the cameras to convey their own images of community problems and strengths.[5] "Participants then work together to select the pictures that best capture their collective wisdom and use these both to tell their stories and to stimulate change through local organizing and institutional—and policy-level action."[8] (*Note:* Needs assessment is discussed in greater length in the second half of this chapter, with regard to program planning.)

Mapping community capacity, on the other hand, is a process of identifying community assets, not concerns or problems. It is a process by which organizers literally use a map to identify the different assets of a community. McKnight and Kretzmann[22] have categorized assets into three different groups based on their availability to the community and refer to them as building blocks. *Primary building blocks* are the most accessible assets. They are located in the neighborhood and are controlled by those who live in the neighborhood. Primary building blocks can be organized into the assets of individuals (e.g., skills and talents) and those of organizations or associations (e.g., religious and citizen organizations). The next most accessible building blocks are secondary building blocks. *Secondary building blocks* are assets located in the neighborhood but largely controlled by people outside (e.g., social service agencies, schools, hospitals, and housing structures). The least accessible assets are referred to as potential building blocks. *Potential building blocks* are resources originating outside the neighborhood and controlled by people outside (e.g., welfare expenditures and public information). By knowing both the needs and assets of the community, organizers can work to identify the true concerns or problems of the community and use the assets of the community as a foundation for dealing with the concerns or problems.

Determining the Priorities and Setting Goals

An analysis of the community assessment data should result in the identification of the problems to be addressed. However, more often than not, the resources needed to solve all identified problems are not available. Therefore, the problems that have been identified must be prioritized. This prioritization is best achieved through general agreement or consensus of those who have been organized so that "ownership" can take hold. It is critical that all those working with the process feel that they "own" the problem and want to see it solved. Without this sense of ownership, they will be unwilling to give of their time and energy to solve it. For example, if a few highly vocal participants intimidate people into voting for certain activities to be the top priorities before a consensus is actually reached, it is unlikely that those who disagreed on this assignment of priorities will work enthusiastically to help solve the problem. They may even drop out of the process because they feel they have no ownership in the decision-making process.

Miller (as cited in Minkler and Wallenstein[5]) has identified five criteria that community organizers need to consider when selecting a priority issue or problem. The issue or problem (1) must be winnable, ensuring that working on it does not simply reinforce fatalistic attitudes and beliefs that things cannot be improved; (2) must be simple and specific, so that any member of the organizing group can explain it clearly in a sentence or two; (3) must unite members of the organizing group and must involve them in a meaningful way in achieving resolution of the issue or problem; (4) should affect many people and build up the community; and (5) should be a part of a larger plan or strategy to enhance the community.[27]

Once the problems have been prioritized, goals need to be identified and written that will serve as guides for problem solving. The practice of consensus building should again be employed during the setting of goals. These goals, which will become the foundation for all the work that follows, can be thought of as the "hoped-for end result." In other words, once community action has occurred, what will have changed? In the community where violence is a problem, the goal may be to reduce the number of violent crimes or eliminate them altogether. Sometimes at this point in the process, some members of the larger group drop out because they do not see their priorities or goals included on consensus lists. Unable to feel ownership, they are unwilling to expend their resources on this process. Because there is strength in numbers, efforts should be made to keep them in. One strategy for doing so is to keep the goal list as long as possible.

Arriving at a Solution and Selecting Intervention Strategies

There are alternative solutions for every community problem. The group should examine the alternatives in terms of probable outcomes, acceptability to the community, probable long- and short-term effects on the community, and the cost of resources to solve the problem.[28] A solution involves selecting one or more intervention strategies (see Table 2). Each type of intervention strategy has advantages and disadvantages. The group must try to agree on the best strategy and then select the most advantageous intervention activity or activities. Again, the group must work toward consensus through compromise. If the educators in the group were asked to provide a recommended strategy, they might suggest offering more preventive-education programs; law enforcement personnel might recommend more enforceable laws; judges might want more space in the jails and prisons. The protectionism of the subgroups within the larger group is often referred to as *turfism*. It is not uncommon to have turf struggles when trying to build consensus.

The Final Steps in the Community Organizing/Building Process: Implementing, Evaluating, Maintaining, and Looping Back

The last four steps in this generalized approach to organizing/building a community include implementing the intervention strategy and activities that were selected in the previous step, evaluating the outcomes of the plans of action, maintaining the outcomes over time, and if necessary, going back to a previous step in the process—"looping back"—to modify or restructure the work plan to organize the community.

Implementation of the intervention strategy includes identifying and collecting the necessary resources for implementation and creating the appropriate time line for implementation. Often the resources can be found within a community, and thus horizontal relationships, the interaction of local units with one another, are needed.[29] Other times the resources

Table 2
Intervention Strategies and Example Activities

1. *Health communication strategies:* Mass media, billboards, booklets, bulletin boards, flyers, direct mail, newsletters, pamphlets, posters, and video and audio materials
2. *Health education strategies:* Educational methods (such as lecture, discussion, and group work) as well as audiovisual materials, computerized instruction, laboratory exercises, and written materials (books and periodicals)
3. *Health policy/enforcement strategies:* Executive orders, laws, ordinances, policies, position statements, regulations, and formal and informal rules
4. *Environmental change strategies:* Those that are designed to change the structure of services or systems of care to improve health promotion services, such as safety belts and air bags in cars, speed bumps in parking lots, or environmental cues such as No Smoking signs
5. *Health-related community services:* The use of health risk appraisals (HRAs), community screening for health problems, and immunization clinics
6. Other strategies
   a. *Behavior modification activities:* Modifying behavior to stop smoking, start to exercise, manage stress, and regulate diet
   b. *Community advocacy activities:* Mass mobilization, social action, community planning, community service development, community education, and community advocacy (such as a letter-writing campaign)
   c. *Organizational culture activities:* Activities that work to change norms and traditions
   d. *Incentives and disincentives:* Items that can either encourage or discourage people to behave a certain way, which may include money and other material items or fines
   e. *Social intervention activities:* Support groups, social activities, and social networks
   f. *Technology-delivered activities:* Educating or informing people by using technology (e.g., computers and telephones)

Source: Adapted from McKenzie, J. F., B. L. Neiger, and R. Thackeray (2009). *Planning, Implementing, and Evaluating Health Promotion Programs: A Primer,* 5th ed. San Francisco, CA: Benjamin Cummings, 201–225.

must be obtained from units located outside the community; in this case, vertical relationships, those where local units interact with extracommunity systems, are needed.[29] An example of this latter relationship is the interaction "between a local nonprofit organization and a state agency with which it has contact."[21]

Evaluation of the process often involves comparing the long-term health and social outcomes of the process to the goals that were set in an earlier step. Some scholars[8] have indicated that such traditional evaluations of community organizing efforts are not easy to carry out and have some limitations. There are times when evaluations are not well planned or funded. As such they "may fail to capture the shorter-term, system-level effects with which community organizing is heavily concerned, such as improvements in organizational collaboration, community involvement, capacity, and healthier public policies or environments.

Maintaining or sustaining the outcomes may be one of the most difficult steps in the entire process. It is at this point that organizers need to seriously consider the need for a long-term capacity for problem solving. Finally, through the steps of implementation, evaluation, and maintenance of the outcomes, organizers may see the need to "loop back" to a previous step in the process to rethink or rework before proceeding onward in their plan.

A Special Note about Community Organizing/Building

Before we leave the processes of community organizing/building, it should be noted that no matter what approach is used in organizing/building a community—locality development, social planning, social action, or the generalized approach outlined here—not all problems can be solved. In other cases, repeated attempts may be necessary before a solution is reached. In addition, it is important to remember that if a problem exists in a community, there are probably some people who benefit from its existence and who may work toward preventing a successful solution to the problem. Whether or not the problem is solved, the final decision facing the organized group is whether to disband the group or to reorganize in order to take on a new problem or attack the first problem from a different direction.

Health Promotion Programming

We discuss how communities describe, analyze, and intervene to solve existing health problems such as disease outbreaks or other community problems. However, the 1979 Surgeon General's report on health promotion and disease prevention, *Healthy People* (see Figure 5), charted a new course for community health—away from curing diseases and toward preventing diseases and promoting health. Health promotion programming has now become an important tool of community health professionals. The second half of this chapter presents the process of health promotion programming.

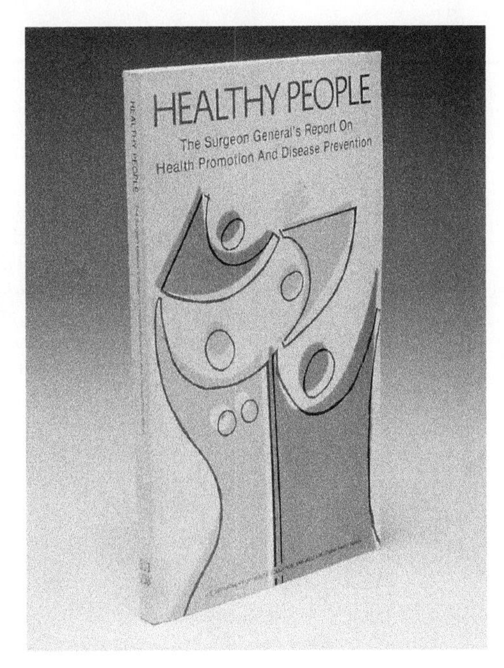

FIGURE 5
Healthy People, the 1979 Surgeon General's report on health promotion and disease prevention, charted a new course for community health.

Basic Understanding of Program Planning

Prior to discussing the process of program planning, two relationships must be presented. These are the relationships between health education and health promotion, and program planning and community organizing/building.

Health education and *health promotion* are terms that are sometimes used interchangeably. This is incorrect because health

health education any combination of planned learning experiences based on sound theories that provide individuals, groups, and communities the opportunity to acquire information and the skills to make quality health decisions

health promotion any planned combination of educational, political, environmental, regulatory, or organizational mechanisms that support actions and conditions of living conducive to the health of individuals, groups, and communities

program planning a process by which an intervention is planned to help meet the needs of a priority population

education is only a part of health promotion. The Joint Committee on Health Education and Promotion Terminology defined the process of **health education** as "any combination of planned learning experiences based on sound theories that provide individuals, groups, and communities the opportunity to acquire information and the skills to make quality health decisions."[30] The committee defined **health promotion** as "any planned combination of educational, political, environmental, regulatory, or organizational mechanisms that support actions and conditions of living conducive to the health of individuals, groups, and communities."[30] From these definitions, it is obvious that the terms are not the same and that *health promotion* is a much more encompassing term than *health education.* Figure 6 provides a graphic representation of the relationship between the terms.

The first half of this chapter described the process of community organizing/building—the process by which individuals, groups, and organizations engage in planned action to influence social problems. Program planning may or may not be associated with community organizing/building. **Program planning** is a process in which an intervention is planned to help meet the needs of a specific group of people. It may take a community organizing/building effort to be able to plan such an intervention. The antiviolence campaign used earlier in the chapter is such an example, where many resources of the community were brought together to create interventions (programs) to deal with the violence problem. However, program planning need not be connected to community organizing/building. For example, a community organizing/building effort is not needed before a company offers a smoking cessation program for its employees or a religious organization offers a stress management class for its members. In such cases, only the steps of the program planning process need to be carried out. These steps are described in the following section.

Creating a Health Promotion Program

The process of developing a health promotion program, like the process of community organizing/building, involves a series of steps. Success depends on many factors, including the assistance of a professional experienced in program planning.

Experienced program planners use models to guide their work. Planning models are the means by which structure and organization are given to the planning process. Many different planning models exist, some of which are used more often than others. Some of the more frequently used models include the PRECEDE/PROCEED model,[31] probably the best known and most often used; the Multilevel Approach to Community Health (MATCH),[32] Intervention Mapping,[33] and the more recently developed consumer-based planning models that are based on health communication and social marketing such as CDCynergy[34] and Social Marketing Assessment and Response Tool (SMART).[35] Each of these planning models has its strengths and weaknesses, and each has distinctive components that make it unique. In addition, each of the models has been used to plan health promotion programs in a variety of settings, with many successes.

It is not absolutely necessary that the student studying community health for the first time have a thorough understanding of the models mentioned here, but it is important to know the basic steps in the planning process. Therefore, we present a generalized program development model[13] that draws on the major components of these other models. The steps of this generalized model are presented in Figure 7 and explained in the following paragraphs.

Prior to undertaking the first step in the generalized model it is important to understand the community and engage the **priority population (audience)**, those whom the health promotion program is intended to serve. Understanding the community means finding out as much as possible about the priority population and the environment in which it exists. Engaging the priority population means getting those in the population involved in the early stages of the health promotion program planning process. If the priority population was composed of the employees of a corporation, the planners would want to read all the material they could find about the company, spend time talking with various individuals and subgroups in the company (e.g., new employees, employees who had been with the company for a long time, management, clerical staff, labor representatives) to find out what they wanted from a health promotion program, and review old documents of the company (e.g., health insurance records, labor agreements, written history of the company). Also, the planners should consider forming a program planning committee with representation from the various subgroups of the workforce (i.e., management, labor, and clerical staff). The planning committee can help ensure that all segments of the priority population will be engaged in the planning process.

priority population (audience)
those whom a program is intended to serve

Assessing the Needs of the Priority Population

needs assessment the process of collecting and analyzing information, to develop an understanding of the issues, resources, and constraints of the priority population, as related to the development of the health promotion program

To create a useful and effective program for the priority population, planners, with the assistance of the planning committee, must determine the needs and wants of the priority population. This procedural step is referred to as a *needs assessment.* A **needs assessment** is the process of collecting and analyzing information to develop an understanding of the issues, resources, and constraints of the priority population, as related to the development of the health promotion program.[36] The assessment's purpose is to determine whether the needs of the people are being met.

For those interested in a detailed explanation of the process of conducting a needs assessment, extensive accounts are available.[37,38] The following is a simplified six-step approach.[13]

Step 1: Determining the Purpose and Scope of the Needs Assessment

The first step in the needs assessment process is to determine the purpose and the scope of the needs assessment. That is, what is the goal of the needs assessment? What does the planning committee hope to gain from the needs assessment? How extensive will the assessment be? What kind of resources will be available to conduct the needs assessment? Once these questions are answered, the planners are ready to begin gathering data.

Step 2: Gathering Data

The second step in the process is gathering the data that will help to identify the true needs of the priority population. Such data are categorized into two groups—primary and secondary. Primary data are those that are collected specifically for use in this process. An example is having those in the priority population complete a needs assessment questionnaire about their health behavior. The completion of the questionnaire may be in a traditional paper-pencil format, as an online survey, or via face-to-face or telephone interviews (see Figure 8). Secondary data are data that have already been collected for some other purpose, such as health insurance claims records or Behavioral Risk Factor Surveillance System (BRFSS) data. Using both primary and secondary data usually presents the clearest picture of the priority population's needs.

Step 3: Analyzing the Data

Collected data can be analyzed in one of two ways—formally or informally. Formal analysis consists of some type of statistical analysis, assuming that the appropriate statistical criteria have been met. However, a more common means of analysis is an informal technique referred to as "eyeballing the data." With this technique, program planners look for the obvious differences between the health status or conditions of the priority population and the programs and services available to close the gap between what is and what ought to be. Regardless of the method used, data analysis should yield a list of the problems that exist, with a description of the nature and extent of each.

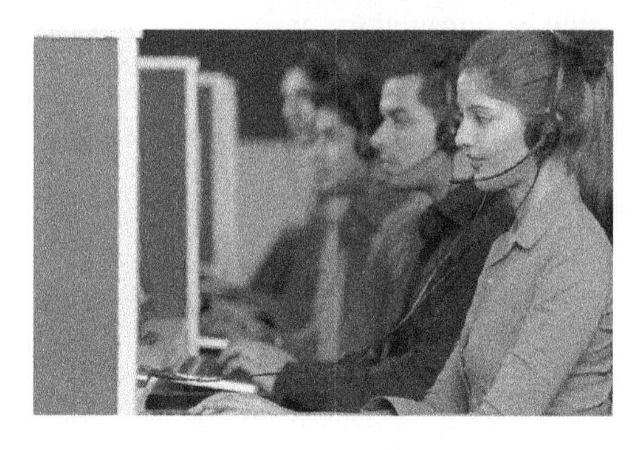

FIGURE 8
A telephone survey is a common form of data collection for a health needs assessment.

The final part of this step is prioritizing the list of problems. Prioritization must take place because though all needs are important, seldom are there enough resources (money and time) available to deal with all the problems identified. When prioritizing, planners should consider (1) the importance of the need, (2) how changeable the need is, and (3) whether adequate resources are available to deal with the problem.

Step 4: Identifying the Factors Linked to the Health Problem

In this step of the process, planners need to identify and prioritize the risk factors that are associated with the health problem. Thus, if the prioritized health problem identified in step 3 is heart disease, planners must analyze the health behaviors and environment of the priority population for known risk factors of heart disease. For example, higher than expected smoking behavior may be present in the priority population in addition to a community that lacks recreational areas for exercise. Once these risk factors are identified, they also need to be prioritized.

Step 5: Identifying the Program Focus

With risk factors identified and prioritized, planners need to identify those *predisposing*, *enabling*, and *reinforcing* factors that seem to have a direct impact on the targeted risk factors. In the heart disease example, those in the priority population may not (1) have the knowledge to begin an exercise program (predisposing factor), (2) have access to recreational facilities (enabling factor), or (3) have people around them who value the benefits of exercise (reinforcing factor). Once the predisposing, enabling, and reinforcing factors have been identified, they too need to be prioritized. As in step 2 earlier, planners can prioritize these factors according to their importance and changeability.[31] The resulting prioritized list provides the program focus.

Step 6: Validating the Prioritized Need

The final step in this process is to double-check or to confirm that the identified need and resulting program focus indeed need to be addressed in the priority population. For example, a limited amount of data may indicate the primary need of the priority group to be one thing—knowledge about heart disease, for example. However, more extensive data or more comprehensive networking may identify another problem such as lack of free or inexpensive recreational facilities. Before step 6 is completed, planners must make sure they have indeed identified a true need. In short, all work should be double-checked.

At the conclusion of a needs assessment, planners should be able to answer the following questions:[38]

1. Who is the priority population?
2. What are the needs of the priority population?
3. Which subgroups within the priority population have the greatest need?
4. Where are the subgroups located geographically?
5. What is currently being done to resolve identified needs?
6. How well have the identified needs been addressed in the past?

Setting Appropriate Goals and Objectives

Once the problem has been well defined and the needs prioritized, the planners can set goals and develop objectives for the program. The goals and objectives should be thought of as the foundation of the program and for the evaluation. The remaining portions of the programming process—intervention development, implementation, and evaluation—will be designed to achieve the goals by meeting the objectives.

The words *goals* and *objectives* are often used interchangeably, but there is really a significant difference between the two. "A goal is a future event toward which a committed endeavor is directed; objectives are the steps taken in pursuit of a goal."[39] To further distinguish between goals and objectives, McKenzie and colleagues[13] have stated that goals (1) are much more encompassing and global than objectives, (2) are written to cover all aspects of a program, (3) provide overall program direction, (4) are more general in nature, (5) usually take longer to complete, (6) do not have a deadline, (7) are usually not observed but inferred,[40] and (8) often not measured in exact terms. Goals are easy to write and include two basic components—who will be affected and what will change because of the program. Here are some examples of program goals:

1. To help employees learn how to manage their stress
2. To reduce the number of teenage pregnancies in the community
3. To help cardiac patients and their families deal with the lifestyle changes that occur after a heart attack

Objectives are more precise and, as noted earlier, can be considered the steps to achieve the program goals. Because some program goals are more complex than others, the number and type of objectives will vary from program to program. For example, the process of getting a group of people to exercise is a more complex activity than trying to get a group to learn the four food groups. The more complex a program, the greater the number of objectives needed. To deal with these different types of programs, McKenzie and colleagues[13] adapted a hierarchy of program objectives first developed by Deeds[41] and later updated by Cleary and Neiger.[42] Table 3 presents the hierarchy and an example of an objective at each of the levels within the hierarchy.

From the examples presented in Table 3, it should be obvious that the hierarchy goes from less complex to more complex levels. Thus, it takes less energy and fewer resources to increase awareness in the priority population than to improve its health status. Close examination of the example objectives reveals that the objectives are written in specific terms. They are composed of four parts (who, what, when, and how much) and outline changes

Table 3
Hierarchy of Objectives and Examples of Each

Type of Objective	Program Outcomes	Possible Evaluation Measures	Type of Evaluation	Example Objective
Process objectives	Activities presented and tasks completed	Number of sessions held, exposure, attendance, participation, staff performance, appropriate materials, adequacy of resources, tasks on schedule	Process (form of formative)	On June 12, 2011, a breast cancer brochure will be distributed to all female customers over the age of 18 at the Ross grocery store.
Impact objectives				
Learning objectives	Change in awareness, knowledge, attitudes, and skills	Increase in awareness, knowledge, attitudes, and skill development/acquisition	Impact (form of summative)	When asked in class, 50% of the students will be able to list the four principles of cardiovascular conditioning.
Action/behavioral objectives	Change in behavior	Current behavior modified or discontinued, or new behavior adopted	Impact (form of summative)	During a telephone interview, 35% of the residents will report having had their blood cholesterol checked in the last 6 months.
Environmental objectives	Change in the environment	Measures associated with economic, service, physical, social, psychological, or political environments, e.g., protection added to, or hazards or barriers removed from, the environment	Impact (form of summative)	By the end of the year, all senior citizens who requested transportation to the congregate meals will have received it.
Outcome objectives	Change in quality of life (QOL), health status, or risk, and social benefits	QOL measures, morbidity data, mortality data, measures of risk (e.g., HRA)	Outcome (form of summative)	By the year 2015, infant mortality rates will be reduced to no more than 7 per 1,000 in Franklin County.

Source: Adapted from Deeds, S. G. (1992). *The Health Education Specialist: Self-Study for Professional Competence.* Los Alamitos, CA: Loose Cannon; Cleary, M. J., and B. L. Neiger (1998). *The Certified Health Education Specialist: A Self-Study Guide for Professional Competence*, 3rd ed. Allentown, PA: National Commission for Health Education Credentialing; and McKenzie, J. F., B. L. Neiger, and R. Thackeray (2009). *Planning, Implementing, and Evaluating Health Promotion Programs: A Primer*, 5th ed. San Francisco, CA: Benjamin Cummings.

BOX 1

HEALTHY PEOPLE 2020: OBJECTIVES

Educational and Community-Based Programs

Goal: Increase the quality, availability, and effectiveness of educational and community-based programs designed to prevent disease and injury, improve health, and enhance quality of life.

Objective: ECBP-10 Increase the number of community-based organizations (including local health departments, tribal health services, nongovernmental organizations, and state agencies) providing population-based primary prevention services in the following areas:

ECBP 10.8 Nutrition

Target: 94.7 percent.

Baseline: 86.4 percent of community-based organizations (including local health departments, tribal health services, nongovernmental organizations, and state agencies) provided population-based primary prevention services in nutrition in 2008.

Target setting method: 10 percent improvement.

Data source: National Profile of Local Health Departments, National Association of County and City Health Officials (NACCHO)

ECBP 10.9 Physical Activity

Target: 88.5 percent.

Baseline: 80.5 percent of community-based organizations (including local health departments, tribal health services, nongovernmental organizations, and State agencies) provided population-based primary prevention services in physical activity in 2008.

Target setting method: 10 percent improvement.

Data source: National Profile of Local Health Departments, National Association of County and City Health Officials (NACCHO).

Note: Other areas covered by this objective include: 10.1 Injury, 10.2 Violence, 10.3 Mental Illness, 10.4 Tobacco Use, 10.5 Substance Abuse, and 10.6 Unintended Pregnancy, and 10.7 Chronic Diseases Programs.

For Further Thought

If you had the opportunity to write one more objective dealing with the implementation of health promotion programs for use in *Healthy People 2020*, what would it be? What is your rationale for selecting such an objective?

Source: U.S. Department of Health and Human Services, Office of Disease Prevention and Health Promotion (2010). *Healthy People 2020*. Available at http://www.healthypeople.gov/2020/default.aspx. Accessed January 4, 2011.

that should result from the implementation of the program.[43] As such, the objectives are written so that the level of their attainment is observable and measurable.

One final note about objectives: *Healthy People 2020,* the national health goals and objectives of the nation, was discussed. Selected objectives from this publication are presented in boxes throughout this text (see Box 1). These goals and objectives provide a good model for developing goals and objectives for a new program. In fact, these goals and objectives can be adapted for use in most community health promotion programs.

Creating an Intervention That Considers the Peculiarities of the Setting

The next step in the program planning process is to design activities that will help the priority population meet the objectives and, in the process, achieve the program goals. These activities are collectively referred to as an **intervention**, or treatment. This intervention or treatment constitutes the program that the priority population will experience.

intervention an activity or activities designed to create change in people

The number of activities in an intervention may be many or only a few. Although no minimum number has been established, it has been shown that multiple activities are often more effective than a single activity. For example, if the planners wanted to change the attitudes of community members toward a new landfill, they would have a greater chance of doing so by distributing pamphlets door to door, writing articles for the local newspaper, and speaking to local service groups, than by performing any one of these activities by itself. In other words, the size and amount of intervention are important in health promotion programming. Few people change their behavior based on a single exposure; instead, multiple exposures are generally needed to change most behaviors. It stands to reason that "hitting" the priority population from several angles or through multiple channels should increase the chances of making an impact.[13]

multiplicity
the number of activities that make up the intervention

dose
the number of program units as part of the intervention

Two terms that relate to the size and amount of an intervention are *multiplicity* and *dose*. **Multiplicity** refers to the number of activities that make up the intervention, while **dose** refers to the number of program units delivered. Thus, if an intervention has two activities—say, an educational workshop and a public service announcement for radio—they define multiplicity, while the number of times each of the activities is presented defines the dose.[13]

best practices
recommendations for interventions based on critical review of multiple research and evaluation studies that substantiate the efficacy of the intervention

The actual creation of the intervention should begin by asking and answering a series of questions.[13] The first is, what needs to change? The answer to this question comes from the needs assessment and the resulting goals and objectives. The second question is, at what level of prevention (i.e., primary, secondary, or tertiary) will the program be aimed? The approach taken to a primary prevention need, that is, preventing a problem before it begins, would be different from a tertiary prevention need of managing a problem after it has existed for a while. The third question asks, at what level of influence will the intervention be focused? The various levels of influence (i.e., intrapersonal, interpersonal, institutional or organizational, community, and public policy) that were presented at the beginning of the chapter as part of the social ecological approach need to be considered. These levels provide the planners with a framework from which to think about how they will "attack" the needs of the priority population. For example, if the goal of a program is to reduce the prevalence of smoking in a community, the intervention could attack the problem by focusing the intervention on individuals through one-on-one counseling, via groups by offering smoking cessation classes, by trying to change policy by enacting a state law prohibiting smoking in public places, or by attacking the problem using more than one of these strategies.

best experience
intervention strategies used in prior or existing programs that have not gone through the critical research and evaluation studies and thus fall short of best practice criteria

The fourth question asks, has an effective intervention strategy to deal with the focus of the problem already been created? Three sources of guidance for selecting intervention strategies (see Table 2 for a list of strategies)—*best practices, best experiences,* and *best processes.* [31] **Best practices** refers to "recommendations for an intervention, based on critical review of multiple research and evaluation studies that substantiate the efficacy of the intervention in the populations and circumstances in which the studies were done, if not its effectiveness in other populations and situations where it might be implemented."[31] Examples of best practices related to health promotion programs are provided in *The Community Guide: What Works to Promote Health*[44] (see Community Health on the Web at the end of this chapter).

best processes
original intervention strategies that the planners create based on their knowledge and skills of good planning processes including the involvement of those in the priority population and the use of theories and models

When best practice recommendations are not available for use, planners need to look for information on best experiences. **Best experience** intervention strategies are those of prior or existing programs that have not gone through the critical research and evaluation studies and thus fall short of best practice criteria but nonetheless show promise in being effective. Best experiences can often be found by networking with others professionals and by reviewing the literature.

If neither best practices nor best experiences are available to planners, then the third source of guidance for selecting an intervention strategy is using best processes. **Best processes** intervention strategies are original interventions that the planners create based on their knowledge and skills of good planning processes including the involvement of those in the priority population and the theories and models used to change behaviors such as social cognitive theory[45] or the transtheoretical model.[46]

The fifth question asks, is the intervention an appropriate fit for the priority population? In other words, does the planned intervention meet the specific characteristics of the priority population such as the educational level, developmental stages, or the specific cultural characteristics of the people being served?

The sixth, and/final, question that needs to be asked is, are the resources available to implement the intervention selected? Planners need to evaluate the amount of money, time, personnel, and/or space that is needed to carry out the various interventions and make a determination if such resources are available to implement the intervention.

Once all of these questions have been asked and answered the planners can then decide which intervention would be best for the priority population with whom they are working. The general intervention strategies presented in Table 2 associated with community organizing/building are the same ones that planners can use with health promotion interventions.

Implementing the Intervention

The moment of truth is when the intervention is implemented. **Implementation** is the actual carrying out or putting into practice the activity or activities that make up the intervention. More formally, implementation has been defined as "the act of converting planning, goals, and objectives into action through administrative structure, management activities, policies, procedures, regulations, and organizational actions of new programs."[47] It is at this point that the planners will learn whether the product (intervention) they developed will be useful in producing the measurable changes as outlined in the objectives.

implementation
putting a planned program into action

To ensure a smooth-flowing implementation of the intervention, it is wise to pilot test it at least once and sometimes more. A **pilot test** is a trial run. It is when the intervention is presented to just a few individuals who are either from the intended priority population or from a very similar population. For example, if the intervention is being developed for fifth graders in a particular school, it might be pilot tested on fifth graders with similar educational backgrounds and demographic characteristics but from a different school.

pilot test
a trial run of an intervention

The purpose of pilot testing an intervention is to determine whether there are any problems with it. Some of the more common problems that pop up are those dealing with the design or delivery of the intervention; however, any part of it could be flawed. For example, it could be determined during pilot testing that there is a lack of resources to carry out the intervention as planned or that those implementing the intervention need more training. When minor flaws are detected and corrected easily, the intervention is then ready for full implementation. However, if a major problem surfaces—one that requires much time and many resources to correct—it is recommended that the intervention be pilot tested again with the improvements in place before implementation.

An integral part of the piloting process is collecting feedback from those in the pilot group. By surveying the pilot group, planners can identify popular and unpopular aspects of the intervention, how the intervention might be changed or improved, and whether the program activities were effective. This information can be useful in fine-tuning this intervention or in developing future programs.

Once the intervention has been pilot tested and corrected as necessary, it is ready to be disseminated and implemented. If the planned program is being implemented with a large priority population and there is a lot at stake with the implementation, it is advisable that the intervention be implemented gradually rather than all at once. One way of doing so is by phasing in the intervention. **Phasing in** refers to a step-by-step implementation in which the

phasing in
implementation of an intervention with a series of small groups instead of the entire population

intervention is introduced first to smaller groups instead of the entire priority population. Common criteria used for selecting participating groups for phasing in include participant ability, number of participants, program offerings, and program location.[13]

The following is an example of phasing in by location. Assume that a local health department wants to provide smoking cessation programs for all the smokers in the community (priority population). Instead of initiating one big intervention for all, planners could divide the priority population by residence location. Facilitators would begin implementation by offering the smoking cessation classes on the south side of town during the first month. During the second month, they would continue the classes on the south side and begin implementation on the west side of town. They would continue to implement this intervention until all sections of the town were included.

evaluation determining the value or worth of an object of interest

Evaluating the Results

standard of acceptability a comparative mandate, value, norm, or group

The final step in the generalized planning model is the evaluation. Although evaluation is the last step in this model, it really takes place in all steps of program planning. It is very important that planning for evaluation occur during the first stages of program development, not just at the end.

Evaluation is the process in which planners determine the value or worth of the object of interest by comparing it against a **standard of acceptability**.[48] Common standards of acceptability include, but are not limited to, mandates (policies, statutes, and laws), values, norms, and comparison/control groups.

formative evaluation the evaluation that is conducted during the planning and implementing processes to improve or refine the program

Evaluation can be categorized further into summative and formative evaluation. **Formative evaluation** is done during the planning and implementing processes to improve or refine the program. For example, validating the needs assessment and pilot testing are both forms of formative evaluation. **Summative evaluation** begins with the development of goals and objectives and is conducted after implementation to determine the program's effect on the priority population. Often, the summative evaluation is broken down into two categories—*impact* and *outcome evaluation*. **Impact evaluation** focuses on immediate observable effects of a program such as changes in awareness, knowledge, attitudes, skills, environmental surroundings, and behavior of those in the priority population, whereas **outcome evaluation** focuses on the end result of the program and is generally measured by improvements in morbidity, mortality, or vital measures of symptoms, signs, or physiologic indicators.[48]

summative evaluation the evaluation that determines the effect of a program on the priority population

Like other steps in the planning model, the evaluation step can be broken down into smaller steps. The mini-steps of evaluation include planning the evaluation, collecting the necessary evaluative data, analyzing the data, and reporting and applying the results.

impact evaluation focuses on immediate observable effects of a program

Planning the Evaluation

As noted earlier, planning for summative evaluation begins with the development of the goals and objectives of the program. These statements put into writing what should happen as a result of the program. Also in this planning mini-step, it should be determined who will evaluate the program—an *internal evaluator* (one who already is involved in the program) or an *external evaluator* (one from outside the program). In addition, this portion of the evaluation process should identify an evaluation design and a time line for carrying out the evaluation.

outcome evaluation focuses on the end result of the program

Collecting the Data

Data collection includes deciding how to collect the data (e.g., with an online survey, from existing records, by observation), determining who will collect them, pilot testing the procedures, and performing the actual data collection.

Analyzing the Data

Once the data are in hand, they must be analyzed and interpreted. Also, it must be decided who will analyze the data and when the analysis is to be completed.

Reporting the Results

Next the evaluation report should be written. Decisions must be made (if they have not been made already) regarding who should write the report, who should receive the report, in what form, and when.

Applying the Results

With the findings in hand, it then must be decided how they will be used. When time, resources, and effort are spent on an evaluation, it is important that the results be useful for reaching a constructive end and for deciding whether to continue or discontinue the program or to alter it in some way.

Chapter Summary

- A knowledge of community organizing and program planning is essential for community health workers whose job it is to promote and protect the health of the community.
- Community organizing is a process through which communities are helped to identify common problems or goals, mobilize resources, and in other ways develop and implement strategies for reaching their goals that they have collectively set.
- Community building is an orientation to community that is strength-based rather than need-based and stresses the identification, nurturing, and celebration of community assets.
- The steps of the general model for community organizing/building include recognizing the issue, gaining entry into the community, organizing the people, assessing the community, determining the priorities and setting goals, arriving at a solution and selecting the intervention strategies, implementing the plan, evaluating the outcomes of the plan of action, maintaining the outcomes in the community, and, if necessary, looping back.
- Program planning is a process in which an intervention is planned to help meet the needs of a priority population (audience).
- The steps in the program planning process include assessing the needs of the priority population, setting

Scenario: Analysis and Response

The town of Kenzington sounds like a good candidate for a community organizing/building effort. Assume that Kenzington is the town in which you now live and you belong to the group that has taken the issue to the city council. Based on what you know about the problem in the scenario and what you know about your town, answer the following questions.

1. What is the real problem?
2. Who do you think the gatekeepers are in the community?
3. What groups of people in the community might be most interested in solving this problem?
4. What groups might have a vested interest in seeing the problem remain unsolved?
5. What interventions would be useful in dealing with the problem?
6. How would you evaluate your efforts to solve the problem?
7. What strategies might you recommend to make the solution lasting?
8. If you were to look for help on the Internet to deal with this problem, what key words would you use to search the Web for help?

appropriate goals and objectives, creating an intervention that considers the peculiarities of the setting, implementing the intervention, and evaluating the results.

Review Questions

1. What is community organizing?
2. What are the assumptions (identified by Ross) under which organizers work when bringing a community together to solve a problem?
3. What is the difference between top-down and grassroots community organizing?
4. What is meant by the term *gatekeepers*? Who would they be in your home community?
5. Identify the steps in the generalized approach to community organizing/building presented in this chapter.
6. What is meant by community building?
7. What is a needs assessment? Why is it important in the health promotion programming process?
8. What are the five major steps in program development?
9. What are the differences between goals and objectives?
10. What are intervention strategies? Provide five examples.
11. What are *best practices, best experiences,* and *best processes*? How are they different?
12. What is meant by the term *pilot testing*? How is it useful when developing an intervention?
13. What is the difference between formative and summative evaluation? What are impact and outcome evaluation?
14. Name and briefly describe the five major components of program evaluation.

Activities

1. From your knowledge of the community in which you live (or from the yellow pages of the telephone book), generate a list of 7 to 10 agencies that might be interested in creating a coalition to deal with community drug problems. Provide a one-sentence rationale for each why it might want to be involved.
2. Ask your instructor if he or she is aware of any community organizing/building efforts in a local community. If you are able to identify such an effort, make an appointment—either by yourself or with some of your classmates—to meet with the person who is leading the effort and ask the following questions:

   What is the problem that faces the community?

   What is the goal of the group?

   What steps have been taken so far to organize/build the community, and what steps are yet to be taken?

   Who is active in the core group?

   Did the group conduct a community assessment?

   What intervention will be/has been used?

   Is it anticipated that the problem will be solved?
3. Using a smoking cessation program, write one program goal and an objective for each of the levels presented in Table 3.
4. Visit a voluntary health agency in your community, either by yourself or with classmates. Ask employees if you may review any of the standard health promotion programs the agency offers to the community. Examine the program materials, locating the five major components of a program development discussed in this chapter. Then, in a two-page paper, summarize your findings.

Community Health on the Web

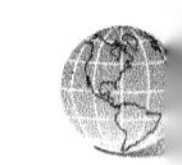

The Internet contains a wealth of information about community and public health. Increase your knowledge of some of the topics presented in this chapter by accessing the Jones & Bartlett Learning Web site at **http://health.jbpub.com/book/communityhealth/7e** and follow the links to complete the following Web activities.

- MAPP
- CDC's Healthy Communities Program
- The Guide to Community Preventive Services

References

1. Rimer, B. K., and K. Glanz (2005). *Theory at a Glance: A Guide for Health Promotion Practice*, 2nd ed. [NIH Pub. No. 05-3896]. Washington, DC: National Cancer Institute.
2. Pellmar, T. C., E. N. Brandt, Jr., and M. Baird (2002). "Health and Behavior: The Interplay of Biological, Behavioral, and Social Influences: Summary of an Institute of Medicine Report." *American Journal of Health Promotion*, 16(4): 206–219.
3. McLeroy, K. R., D. Bibeau, A. Steckler, and K. Glanz (1988). "An Ecological Perspective for Health Promotion Programs." *Health Education Quarterly*, 15(4): 351–378.
4. Sallis, J. F., N. Owen, and E. B. Fisher (2008). "Ecological Models of Health Behavior." In K. Glanz, B. K. Rimer, and K. Viswanath, eds., *Health Behavior and Health Education Practice: Theory, Research, and Practice*, 4th ed. San Francisco, CA: Jossey-Bass, 465–485.
5. Minkler, M., and N. Wallerstein (2005). "Improving Health through Community Organization and Community Building: A Health Education Perspective." In M. Minkler, ed., *Community Organizing and Community Building for Health*, 2nd ed. New Brunswick, NJ: Rutgers University Press, 26–50.
6. Ross, M. G. (1967). *Community Organization: Theory, Principles, and Practice.* New York: Harper and Row, 86–92.

7. Goodman, R. M., M. A. Speers, K. McLeroy, S. Fawcett, M. Kegler, E. Parker, S. R. Smith, T. D. Sterling, and N. Wallerstein (1999). "Identifying and Defining the Dimensions of Community Capacity to Provide a Basis for Measurement." *Health Education and Behavior*, 25(3): 258-278.

8. Minkler, M., N. Wallerstein, and N. Wilson (2008). "Improving Health through Community Organizing and Community Building." In K. Glanz, B. K. Rimer, and K. Viswanath, eds., *Health Behavior and Health Education Practice: Theory, Research, and Practice*, 4th ed. San Francisco, CA: Jossey-Bass, 287-312.

9. Rothman, J., and J. E. Tropman (1987). "Models of Community Organization and Macro Practice Perspectives: Their Mixing and Phasing." In F. M. Cox, J. L. Erlich, J. Rothman, and J. E. Tropman, eds., *Strategies of Community Organization: Macro Practice*. Itasca, IL: Peacock, 3-26.

10. Garvin, C. D., and F. M. Cox (2001). "A History of Community Organizing Since the Civil War with Special Reference to Oppressed Communities." In J. Rothman, J. L. Erlich, and J. E. Tropman, eds., *Strategies of Community Intervention*, 5th ed. Itasca, IL: Peacock, 65-100.

11. Rothman, J. (2001). "Approaches to Community Intervention." In J. Rothman, J. L. Erlich, and J. E. Tropman, eds., *Strategies of Community Intervention*, 6th ed. Itasca, IL: Peacock.

12. Checkoway, B. (1989). "Community Participation for Health Promotion: Prescription for Public Policy." *Wellness Perspectives: Research, Theory, and Practice*, 6(1): 18-26.

13. McKenzie, J. F., B. L. Neiger, and R. Thackeray (2009). *Planning, Implementing, and Evaluating Health Promotion Programs: A Primer*, 5th ed. San Francisco, CA: Benjamin Cummings.

14. Butterfoss, F. D. (2007). *Coalitions and Partnerships in Community Health*. San Francisco, CA: Jossey-Bass.

15. Braithwaite, R. L., F. Murphy, N. Lythcott, and D. S. Blumenthal (1989). "Community Organization and Development for Health Promotion within an Urban Black Community: A Conceptual Model." *Health Education*, 20(5): 56-60.

16. Wright, P. A. (1994). *A Key Step in Developing Prevention Materials Is to Obtain Expert and Gatekeepers' Reviews* (Technical Assistance Bulletin). Bethesda, MD: Center for Substance Abuse Prevention (CASP) Communications Team, 1-6.

17. Tervalon, M., and J. Garcia (1998). "Cultural Humility versus Cultural Competence: A Critical Distinction in Defining Physician Training Outcomes in Multicultural Education." *Journal of Health Care for the Poor and Underserved*, 9(2): 117-125.

18. Perlman, J. (1978). "Grassroots Participation from Neighborhood to Nation." In S. Langton, ed., *Citizen Participation in America*. Lexington, MA: Lexington Books, 65-79.

19. Brager, G., H. Specht, and J. L. Torczyner (1987). *Community Organizing*. New York: Columbia University Press, 55.

20. Minkler, M. (2005). "Introduction to Community Organizing and Community Building." In M. Minkler, ed., *Community Organizing and Community Building for Health*, 2nd ed. New Brunswick, NJ: Rutgers University Press, 1-21.

21. Walter, C. L. (2005). "Community Building Practice: A Conceptual Framework." In M. Minkler, ed., *Community Organizing and Community Building for Health*, 2nd ed. New Brunswick, NJ: Rutgers University Press, 66-78.

22. McKnight, J. L., and J. P. Kretzmann (2005). "Mapping Community Capacity." In M. Minkler, ed., *Community Organizing and Community Building for Health*, 2nd ed. New Brunswick, NJ: Rutgers University Press, 158-172.

23. Hancock, T., and M. Minkler (2005). "Community Health Assessment or Healthy Community Assessment." In M. Minkler, ed., *Community Organizing and Community Building for Health*, 2nd ed. New Brunswick, NJ: Rutgers University Press, 138-157.

24. Nyswander, D. B. (1956). "Education for Health: Some Principles and Their Application." *Health Education Monographs*, 14: 65-70.

25. Wang, C. C., and M. A. Burris (1994). "Empowerment through Photovoice: Portraits of Participation." *Health Education Quarterly*, 21(2): 171-186.

26. Wang, C. C., and M. A. Burris (1997). "Photovoice: Concept, Methodology, and Use for Participatory Needs Assessment." *Health Education and Behavior*, 24(3): 369-387.

27. Miller, M. (1986). "Turning Problems into Actionable Issues." Unpublished paper. San Francisco, CA: Organize Training Center.

28. Archer, S. E., and R. P. Fleshman (1985). *Community Health Nursing*. Monterey, CA: Wadsworth Health Sciences.

29. Warren, R. L. (1963). *The Community in America*. Chicago: Rand-McNally.

30. Joint Committee on Health Education and Promotion Terminology (2001). "Report of the 2000 Joint Committee on Health Education and Promotion Terminology." *American Journal of Health Education*, 32(2): 89-103.

31. Green, L. W., and M. W. Kreuter (2005). *Health Program Planning: An Educational and Ecological Approach*, 4th ed. Boston: McGraw-Hill.

32. Simons-Morton, D. G., W. H. Greene, and N. H. Gottlieb (1995). *Introduction to Health Education and Health Promotion*, 2nd ed. Prospect Heights, IL: Waveland Press.

33. Bartholomew, L. K., G. S. Parcel, G. Kok, and N. H. Gottlieb (2006). *Planning Health Promotion Programs: An Intervention Mapping Approach*, 2nd ed. San Francisco, CA: Jossey-Bass.

34. Centers for Disease Control and Prevention, U.S. Department of Health and Human Services (2003). *CDCynergy 3.0: Your Guide to Effective Health Communication* [CD-ROM Version 3.0]. Atlanta, GA: Author.

35. Neiger, B. L., and R. Thackeray (1998). *Social Marketing: Making Public Health Sense*. Paper presented at the annual meeting of the Utah Public Health Association, Provo, UT.

36. Anspaugh, D. J., M. B. Dignan, and S. L. Anspaugh (2000). *Developing Health Promotion Programs*. Boston: McGraw-Hill Higher Education.

37. Gilmore, G. D., and M. D. Campbell (2005). *Needs and Capacity Assessment Strategies for Health Education and Health Promotion*, 3rd ed. Sudbury, MA: Jones & Bartlett.

38. Peterson, D. J., and G. R. Alexander (2001). *Needs Assessment in Public Health: A Practical Guide for Students and Professionals*. New York, NY: Kluwer Academic/Plenum Publishers.

39. Ross, H. S., and P. R. Mico (1980). *Theory and Practice in Health Education*. Palo Alto, CA: Mayfield, 219.

40. Jacobsen, D., P. Eggen, and D. Kauchak (1989). *Methods for Teaching: A Skills Approach*, 3rd ed. Columbus, OH: Merrill.

41. Deeds, S. G. (1992). *The Health Education Specialist: Self-Study for Professional Competence*. Los Alamitos, CA: Loose Cannon Publications.

42. Cleary, M. J., and B. L. Neiger (1998). *The Certified Health Education Specialist: A Self-Study Guide for Professional Competence*, 3rd ed. Allentown, PA: National Commission for Health Education Credentialing.

43. McKenzie, J. F. (2005). "Planning and Evaluating Interventions." In J. Kerr, R. Weitkunat, and M. Moretti, eds., *ABC of Behavior Change: A Guide to Successful Disease Prevention and Health Promotion*. Oxford, England: Elsevier, 41-54.

44. Centers for Disease Control and Prevention (2010). *Guide to Community Preventive Services—The Community Guide: What Works to Promote Health*. Available at http://www.thecommunityguide.org/index.html.

45. McAlister, A. L., C. L. Perry, and G. S. Parcel (2008). How Individuals, Environments, and Health Behaviors Interact: Social Cognitive Theory. In K. Glanz, B. K. Rimer, and K. Viswanath, eds., *Health Behavior and Health Education: Theory, Research, and Practice*, 4th ed. San Francisco, CA: Jossey-Bass, 167-188.

46. Prochaska, J. O., C. A. Redding, and K. E. Evers (2008). The Transtheoretical Model and Stages of Change. In K. Glanz, B. K. Rimer, and K. Viswanath, eds., *Health Behavior and Health Education: Theory, Research, and Practice*, 4th ed. San Francisco, CA: Jossey-Bass, 97–121.

47. Timmreck, T. C. (1997). *Health Services Cyclopedic Dictionary*, 3rd ed. Sudbury, MA: Jones & Bartlett.

48. Green, L. W., and F. M. Lewis (1986). *Measurement and Evaluation in Health Education and Health Promotion*. Palo Alto, CA: Mayfield.

PHOTO CREDITS

1 © Divanir4a/Dreamstime.com; **4** © Jack Hollingsworth/Photodisc/Getty Images; **5** Courtesy of U.S. Surgeon General's Office; **8** © GoGo Images/age fotostock

Unless otherwise indicated, all photographs and illustrations are under copyright of Jones & Bartlett Learning, or have been provided by the authors.

ndex